A Manual of
Elite Sports and Vision

(An Introduction to Implications of Vision in Sports)

A Manual of *Elite* Sports and Vision

(An Introduction to Implications of Vision in Sports)

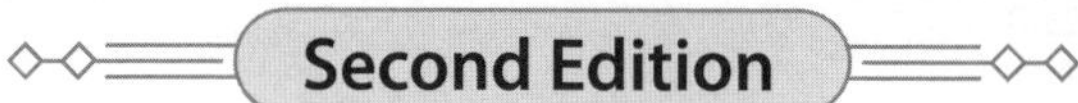

Second Edition

Ajay Kumar Bhootra
B Optom DOS FAO FOAI FCLI ICLEP FIACLE (Australia)
Diploma in Sportvision (UK)
Ex-CEO and Dean
Krishnalaya School of Optometry
Kolkata, West Bengal, India

Sumitra Agarwal
BHMS DMBS MD (Bio) M Optom B Optom DOS
Diploma in Sportvision (UK)
Optometrist, Ocularist and Private Practitioner

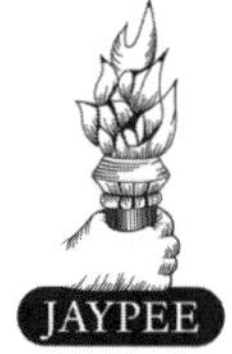

JAYPEE BROTHERS MEDICAL PUBLISHERS
The Health Sciences Publisher
New Delhi | London

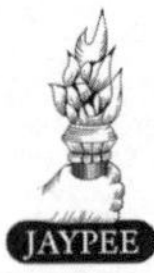

Jaypee Brothers Medical Publishers (P) Ltd

Headquarters
Jaypee Brothers Medical Publishers (P) Ltd
EMCA House, 23/23-B
Ansari Road, Daryaganj
New Delhi 110 002, India
Landline: +91-11-23272143, +91-11-23272703
+91-11-23282021, +91-11-23245672
Email: jaypee@jaypeebrothers.com

Corporate Office
Jaypee Brothers Medical Publishers (P) Ltd
4838/24, Ansari Road, Daryaganj
New Delhi 110 002, India
Phone: +91-11-43574357
Fax: +91-11-43574314
Email: jaypee@jaypeebrothers.com

Overseas Office
J.P. Medical Ltd
83, Victoria Street, London
SW1H 0HW (UK)
Phone: +44 20 3170 8910
Fax: +44 (0)20 3008 6180
Email: info@jpmedpub.com

Website: www.jaypeebrothers.com
Website: www.jaypeedigital.com

Inquiries for bulk sales may be solicited at: jaypee@jaypeebrothers.com

A Manual of Elite Sports and Vision

First Edition: 2008

Second Edition: **2025**

ISBN: 978-93-5696-876-9

Printed in India at Sterling Graphics Pvt. Ltd.

Dedication

A token of respect
to
Mr Geraint Griffiths

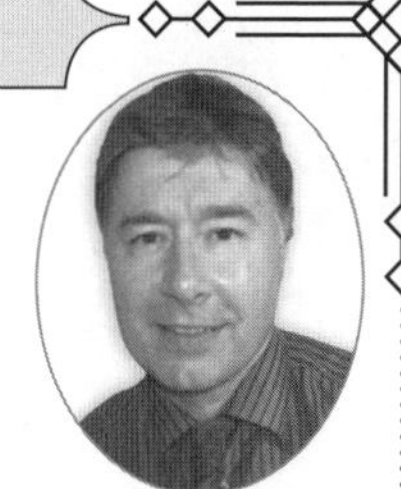

Geraint Griffiths is the founder and CEO of the Association of Sport Vision Practitioners and the author of the Diploma in Sport Vision Practice. As a British College of Optometrists examiner and assessor, and a former British international athlete, Griffiths brings a wealth of expertise to the field of sportvision. His extensive experience and seniority as a researcher in sport vision have greatly influenced the contents of this book, which draws heavily from his teachings.

Preface to the Second Edition

Once upon a time, "business as usual" was often good enough. However, in today's rapidly evolving world, where science fiction is becoming science fact and transforming our businesses and societies daily, "good enough" is no longer sufficient. To thrive, we must excel at driving change rather than being driven by it. As Bill Gates mentioned in his book *Business @ The Speed of Thought*, "Business is going to change more in the next ten years than it has in the last fifty." This statement rings true even in the field of optometry, where we are witnessing significant changes.

When we began our career as an optometrist, patients had simpler needs and limited expectations. Over time, however, this has changed dramatically. Specialization is now in high demand, and patients are well educated, unwilling to settle for anything average. The world of work has been radically reshaped by several forces, leading to a major shift away from the notion of learning one profession, having one job, and staying in it for decades. Embracing a forward-looking practice approach that considers various specializations is critical for professional growth. Sportvision is one such specialization, still in its nascent stage, where the scope and opportunities are immense.

This book is a small effort to reveal the practice secrets of sportvision optometry. The first edition focused on the visual needs in different sports. However, in this edition, we have also included the practice aspects of sportvision optometry. We recognized the need for a concise and accessible book to meet the basic needs of practitioners aspiring to become sportvision specialists. This book will also be a valuable resource for students.

We have organized the contents in an orderly manner, categorizing them for easy reference. Our goal is to provide a comprehensive guide that can be easily referenced as needed.

We hope this book serves as a practical guide and a source of inspiration for those passionate about sportvision optometry.

Ajay Kumar Bhootra
Sumitra Agarwal

Preface to the First Edition

Vision has enormous implications in terms of health and welfare of the nation. Research has shown us in sports that even small visual deficiency in one eye can ruin the game of the athletes. Even more important the same problem can substantially effect everybody's ability to carry out their chosen occupations. Straightforward implication of this is that more important in general terms, because the ability to work efficiently or competing the sport at the highest level is directly related to our vision. Problems with the visual process that are not explained and understood can have profound implications for the athletes and their immediate family and friends. There was no debate about the protection of the eyes from trauma and non-ionizing radiations. But the biggest challenge was to establish the strong scientific basis for understanding the implications of vision in sports. Therefore, researchers established the science of Sportvision in the field of behavioral optometry.

Originally originated in USA, the science actually started to develop in UK under the leadership of Mr Geraint Griffiths since 1994. At the outset, practice began to develop the work already started in USA. But the new researches have given the science a dynamic shape. In India, the science started to flourish at the Himalaya Optical Group where Ajay Kr Bhootra, Optometrist, Ocularist and Diploma in Sportvision (UK) and his colleague Dr Sumitra, BHMS, DMBS, MD, DOS, B.Optom, and Diploma in Sportvision (UK) worked together to explore the implications of sportvision in the field of optometry. The vision in sports has an immediate application to the athletes and in a country that is going through an industrial revolution, it is essential that young talent is not disadvantaged by visual deficiencies. Loss of sporting or occupational performance at any level in society affects general health which ultimately will conspire to decrease the quality of life and life expectancy.

This book is a small effort to reveal the importance of vision in sports and sporting performance of the athletes and is intended for all those who are interested in sports and vision. These may include eyecare professionals including optometrists and ophthalmologists and sports medicine practitioners, sports coaches team managers, sports clubs, sports associations, athletes, players and all those parents who want their kids to excel in sports. The authors do not claim it to be a comprehensive book to include complete information on sportvision practice. It is just an effort to appreciate the immediate need for basic information on the importance of vision in sports as the sports today is no more a recreational activity only. It has become one of the biggest industries where millions of dollars are involved in the form of fees, prizes, advertisements and sponsorships. It is intended that this book will fulfill basic educational requirements, stimulate people's interest in sportvision and provide a reference source. The science of sportvision is still new and the results of many researches will follow. Ideas about the role of vision in different sports may vary depending upon the level of sports and accessibility to the new researches. Hence, readers are strongly encouraged to keep themselves up-to-date and help establish the science of sportvision as an accepted discipline by providing us their opinions.

Ajay Kumar Bhootra
Sumitra Agarwal

Acknowledgements

Writing a book is not a solitary endeavor; it is a collaborative journey enriched by the support, encouragement, and contributions of many individuals. As we pen down these words of acknowledgment, we extend our deepest gratitude to those whose presence and efforts have shaped this work.

First and foremost, we express our heartfelt thanks to our family for their unwavering support and understanding during the countless hours spent immersed in research and writing.

We are grateful to our mentors and advisors, whose guidance has been invaluable. Their wisdom, constructive feedback, and expert insights have played a pivotal role in shaping the content of this book.

I am very grateful to the whole team of M/s Jaypee Brothers Medical Publishers (P) Ltd, New Delhi, India, who helped and guided me, Shri Jitendar P Vij (Group Chairman), Mr Ankit Vij (Managing Director), Mr MS Mani (Group President), Dr Madhu Choudhary (Director–Educational Publishing), Ms Pooja Bhandari [Director–Production (Books and Journals)], Mr Ajay Kumar Sharma [Deputy General Manager (Books and Journals)], Ms Sunita Katla (Executive Assistant to Group Chairman and Publishing Manager), Ms Samina Khan (Executive Assistant to Director–Educational Publishing), Dr Upma Tomar (Senior Development Editor), Mr Rajesh Sharma (Production Coordinator), Ms Seema Dogra (Cover Visualizer), Ms Neha Verma (Graphic Designer–Cover), Ms Neelam Kakriya (Proofreader), Mr Deep Kumar (Typesetter), Mr Rajesh Ghurkundi (Graphic Designer) and their team members, for all their support to work in this project and make it a success. Without their cooperation, I could not have completed this project.

Last but not least, we extend our gratitude to the readers. We hope the pages ahead offer insights, inspiration, and a meaningful contribution to the subject matter.

With gratitude!

Ajay Kumar Bhootra
Sumitra Agarwal

Contents

Sports: An Occupation

1 CHAPTER

Play plays a crucial role in the holistic development of a child, contributing to both their emotional and physical well-being. Playing activities foster the development of fundamental motor skills such as climbing, walking, jumping, and hand-eye coordination through activities like throwing and catching. As play evolves and begins to incorporate rules, it transforms into structured games and sports, fostering individual and team participation.

When the play begins to incorporate rules, it becomes a game leading to sports with both individual and team participations. The word 'sport' is a contracted form of "disport" which means to amuse, to divert one's self. It signifies recreations that are contrasted with the serious intellectual occupations.

Tennis, classified as an individual sport, and football, a team sport, represent the pinnacle of organized activities guided by specific rules. In both, mental preparation is crucial as players strategically navigate their respective fields, whether it is a tennis court or a football pitch. Success in these sports hinges on a blend of physical proficiency, disciplined training, and a commitment to following established rules. The competitive nature of both sports sets them apart, demanding a strategic mindset and a dedication to achieving goals, whether individually or collectively. In essence, these sports showcase the harmonious interplay between individual skills and teamwork, making them dynamic and multifaceted endeavors.

The term 'sport' can be defined as a competitive activity, whether against others or oneself. The competitive element becomes a defining characteristic, setting sports apart from mere physical activities. This competitive aspect, whether in team sports like football or individual pursuits, serves as a notable differentiator. In essence, sports encompass a broad spectrum of activities that involve competition, combining physical exertion with strategic planning. Whether played individually or in teams, the rules and objectives provide structure, turning play into a more organized and purposeful pursuit.

Sports constitute organized, structured, and competitive physical activities governed by defined rules. Involving two or more players, these activities aim to determine a clear winner or loser, sometimes resulting in a draw that may be settled through mechanisms like penalty shoot-outs. At the elite level, sports demand intense competition and rigorous physical, emotional, and mental training.

Success at the elite level is not the same as talent. The world is full of incredible, talented athletes and players who struggled in their lives to succeed. Talent usually does not lead to differentiation at the elite level. It is the training, preparations, or individual commitment that makes or breaks at this level. One has to constantly look for extra gear, which means there is no room for putting a smiley face on what you do. Most players at this level also spend a sufficient amount of time on training and preparations, which has created a situation where it has become difficult to differentiate between a good player and a great player. This is why most athletes at this level look for one elusive factor that would give them an extra edge over their competitors. Vision can often be one such elusive factor because sporting performance is strongly related to visual performance. Many experts say that at the elite level, the athlete, in fact, doesn't compete with anyone. They constantly look for their opponent's weakness and attack. They see the situation, their killer instinct kicks in, and they attack. This is not easy. It takes tireless dedication and consistent hard work in every aspect of training because one missed opportunity at the elite level may prove to be a career-ending event.

Sport is about a calm mind and a violent body. It is difficult to stay calm amidst the pressure to perform. The idea is to get a rush, a flow of adrenaline, and then to remain calm in the situation. A calm mind is not about doing nothing. It is about keeping oneself busy in the situation and keeping the mind away from other thoughts. When you compete with highly successful and high-profile athletes, there is a saying that you live by yourself or you won't stay for long in that world.

"A sound mind in a sound body" can be thought of through the sports. Athletics refresh the body, tranquilize and enlighten the mind, and develop moral character. They are always fresh and full of energy. They seldom get sick and tired. They are capable of good, positive and free thinking. They have a strong will power and better control on their behavior, sentiments and emotions.

Motivation is probably the strongest incentive, and the concept of "win at all costs" is often initiated. The incentive to win may vary from personal satisfaction, team spirit, or national fervour to the high monetary awards accorded to professional sports personnel. Aptitude in sports is sometimes influenced by physique. In general, shorter athletes are more suited to events like gymnastics, soccer, and long-distance running; tall individuals predominate in high jumping and basketball, while heavyweights are more likely to be attracted to combat sports like throwing and defensive positions in rugby.

FACTORS THAT AFFECT SPORTING PERFORMANCE

Success in sports is never achieved by chance. A large range of physical and mental factors contribute to the successful performance in sports, some of the important among them are shown in **Figure 1.1**.

Skills

Each sport and activity require a specific set of skills. They may be technical skills and tactical skills. While technical skills are proficiency in the specific

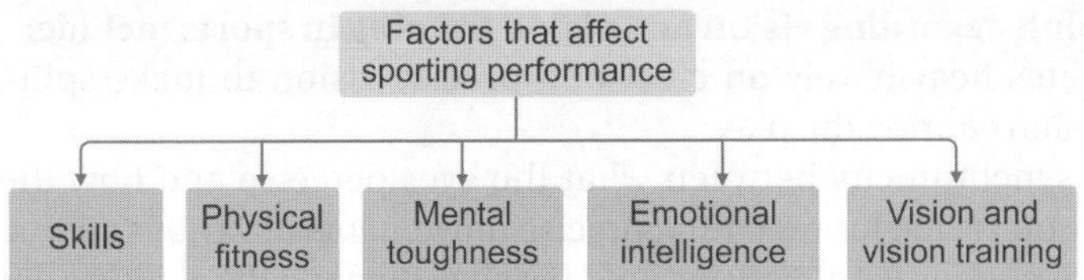

Fig. 1.1: Factors that affect sporting performance.

skills required for the sport is fundamental, tactical skills are understanding and implementing effective strategies during competition. These skills may be innate or acquired and can be optimized by coaching and training. These skills are the most significant formula for success. Being successful in one sport does not necessarily make you successful in another.

Physical Fitness

Fitness plays a major role in success for many sports. Fitness determines the ability to exercise for extended period of time without tiring, ability to move quickly across the grounds or move limbs rapidly to grab or throw.

Mental Toughness

Physical fitness can make an athlete good but mental toughness is what ultimately makes a great athlete. It is difficult to train the body before training the mind. The true measure of an athlete is determined by the factors that are intangibles. Mental resilience is critical for coping with pressure, setbacks, and adapting to unforeseen situations is vital.

Emotional Intelligence

A thorough understanding of emotional intelligence leads to perfecting the mental side of an athlete. This is because traits like persistence, determination, and teamwork become easier to display if the athlete has full control of his emotions. Daniel Goleman, an American psychologist has talked about five main components of emotional intelligence—self-awareness, self-regulation, motivation, empathy and social skills.

Vision and Vision Training

Vision and vision training stand as paramount elements in sports performance, as the ability to see clearly and accurately significantly impacts an athlete's effectiveness in various disciplines. Whether it's tracking a flying ball, returning a serve, making a precision pass, or aiming to hit a target, the eyes play a leading role, guiding the rest of the body in execution. Vision training emerges as a crucial tool to enhance an athlete's visual capabilities, coordination between the two eyes, eye focusing, and eye-hand coordination. By addressing these aspects, vision training aims to reduce reaction time, a key factor in elevating overall sporting performance.

Key points regarding vision and vision training in sports include:

- Athletes heavily rely on clear and precise vision to make split-second decisions during the play.
- The synchronicity between what the eyes perceive and how the hands respond is vital for executing precise movements in various sports.
- Sports such as tennis, cricket, and baseball demand the ability to accurately track and anticipate the trajectory of fast-moving objects, often requiring rapid adjustments.
- Vision training targets improvements in the speed at which an athlete processes visual information and initiates a physical response.
- Ensuring that both eyes work seamlessly together is crucial for depth perception and accurately perceiving the spatial relationships within the sporting environment.
- Tailoring vision training exercises to the specific demands of a particular sport can optimize an athlete's visual skills in that context.
- Peripheral vision is essential in sports where awareness of the entire playing field or court is necessary. Vision training may include exercises to expand and enhance peripheral vision.
- Vision training can improve an athlete's ability to focus on relevant details, filtering out distractions that might affect performance.

Considering the intricate interplay of these factors, optimizing sporting performance often requires a holistic and individualized approach tailored to the athlete's unique characteristics and circumstances.

TYPES OF SPORTS

Sport can be broadly categorized into amateur, professional, and international domains, each characterized by distinct features and organizational structures. However, defining the boundary between amateur and professional athletes can be challenging, as different organizations may have varying criteria. A straightforward yet practical distinction is that amateur athletes engage in sports as a hobby, while professional athletes pursue sports as a career.

The concept of amateur sports encompasses a wide spectrum, ranging from individual recreational activities to high school sports and organized intercollegiate or international competitions. Various groups manage and organize athletic activities, establishing rules for eligibility and competition. These rules help maintain fairness and integrity within the sporting community.

In the realm of professional sports, a pivotal aspect is the contractual relationship between individual players and team owners, governed by fundamental contract principles. The model contract serves as a framework but can be adjusted to accommodate the unique needs and talents of each player. This contractual arrangement is crucial in shaping the dynamics of professional sports, including player transfers, endorsements, and financial agreements.

International sports competitions play a significant role, with events such as the Olympics and the FIFA World Cup standing out as premier examples. These competitions not only showcase athletic prowess on a global stage but also foster international camaraderie. Organizations like FIFA play a central role in organizing and overseeing these events, ensuring adherence to established rules and regulations.

Sports can be classified into two primary categories: dynamic and non-dynamic sports **(Table 1.1)**. Non-dynamic sport is also called controlled sports. In dynamic sports, athletes experience relatively uninhibited and explosive expressions of effort. While control is still essential, the emphasis lies on the explosive elements, serving as a critical differentiator between athletes. Examples of dynamic sports include 100-m running, hammer throwing, soccer, yachting, squash **(Fig. 1.2)**, hockey, among others.

Conversely, non-dynamic sports involve repetitive actions that may extend overextended durations. Success in these sports hinges on maintaining consistent performance throughout the event. In control sports, the athlete's ability to sustain a high level of performance over time is the key to victory.

Table 1.1: Dynamic sports and non-dynamic sports.

Dynamic sports	*Non-dynamic sports*
Soccer	Archery
Yachting	Bowling
Squash	Shooting
Hockey	Dart
Ice-hockey	Snooker
Baseball	Chess

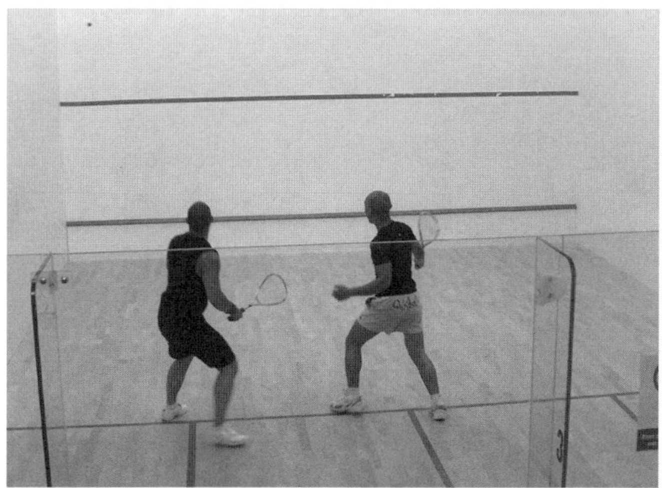

Fig. 1.2: Squash—dynamic sport.

This requires precise physiological control, mitigating factors such as muscle fatigue, dehydration, blood sugar levels, and mental fatigue. The skill in these sports is not merely achieving a perfect shot once, as in hitting the bulls eye or the gold in archery, but rather maintaining unwavering consistency over the entire duration of the competition. **Table 1.1** shows the different types of dynamic and non-dynamic sports.

Neither dynamic sports nor controlled sports can be deemed easier or superior to the other. Water sports, for instance, may lack the speed and explosiveness seen in dynamic sports, but it compensates with microscopic control and endurance. Other examples of controlled sports include archery, bowling, shooting, darts, snooker **(Fig. 1.3)**, and chess. Chess, in particular, stands out as an extreme example where the apparent static nature masks the intense mental equilibrium required. The players maintain a dynamic equilibrium, coordinating their eyes precisely on the chessboard while their minds process a complex image of spatial awareness and position. Despite the lack of physical dynamism, chess demands significant mental effort and is highly competitive.

Fast-moving sports predominantly fall into the dynamic category, allowing for a more precise consideration of hazards and playing speed. However, most sports are a blend of both dynamic and controlled elements in varying proportions. Visual correction considerations evolve as the balance between dynamic and non-dynamic, physical and cerebral aspects of sports shifts. For instance, in high-speed sports like ice hockey and tennis, there is a significant risk of trauma, necessitating quick reactions and visual acuity. Conversely, in chess, with minimal movement and a focus on strategic thinking, the risk of eye injuries is low. Despite these differences, the intensity of competition in both dynamic and controlled sports should not be underestimated. Each type presents its own set of challenges, requiring athletes to excel in diverse skill sets and mental capacities.

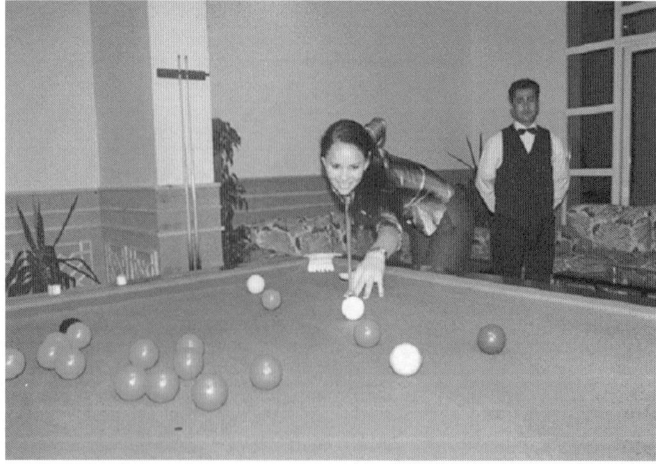

Fig. 1.3: Snooker—non-dynamic sports.

Sports, much like other occupations, come with their own set of requirements, and sporting potential can be viewed as a form of occupational potential. In essence, occupation encompasses how individuals interact with their environment, whether in the workplace, sports, or daily life. This interaction involves specific skills and behaviors, ranging from navigating the world to social interactions and even learning essential skills like reading and writing. In this context, terms like "sporting potential," "occupational potential," and "behavior" can be used interchangeably.

Applying the principles of occupational therapy to sporting performance is a viable approach. Occupational therapy, traditionally associated with improving individuals' ability to engage in daily activities, can be extended to enhance an athlete's performance. This approach places a focus on the athlete's involvement in their chosen sport throughout the evaluation and intervention processes.

During the evaluation phase, attention is given to understanding the athlete's sporting needs, challenges, and aspirations. All aspects of performance are considered equally important for effectiveness during competition. The intervention strategies that follow aim to enhance sporting performance based on the identified needs. The success of these strategies is gauged by assessing whether the desired improvements have been achieved.

Recognizing the critical nature of intervention in sports is essential, as even a momentary lapse can have significant consequences for an athlete. The evaluation and intervention processes in occupational therapy for sports performance are tailored to the specific demands of the chosen sport, emphasizing a holistic approach to enhance overall effectiveness.

Currently, over 60% of the population engages in sports, a trend influenced by increased resources, a rise in financial investments, and individuals having more time and disposable income. This surge in sports participation is underscored by its recognition as a necessity. Notably, the popularity of sports has led to a significant increase in hospital admissions for serious eye injuries, emphasizing its widespread appeal.

In the realm of sports, a fundamental reality is that winners coexist with losers. The champion occupies the pinnacle of a vast pyramid **(Fig. 1.4)**, with spectators, organizers, coaches, clubs, and officials forming the supportive base. Winning is inherently linked to the existence of competitors who may come second or third. The cyclical nature of victories and losses is well understood by competitive athletes; winning one day often means losing another. Recognizing the importance of the collective effort is crucial—

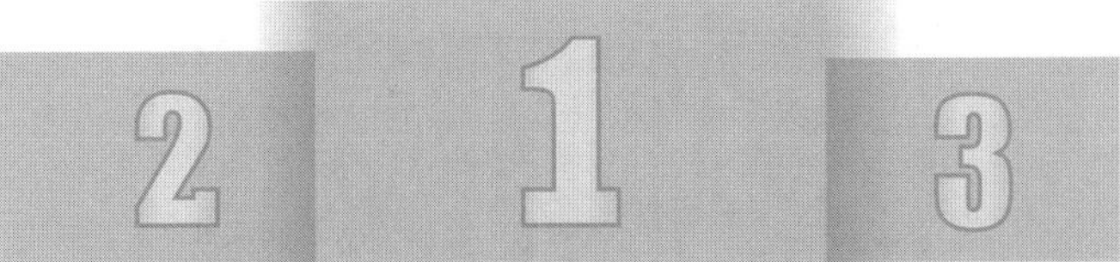

Fig. 1.4: Winning has no meaning unless someone else.

nothing can be achieved without the support of everyone involved in the event, including those willing to accept the possibility of losing.

This interconnectedness echoes a broader truth applicable to life at large. Interdependence is a fundamental aspect of human existence, wherein individuals rely on one another, and nations depend on each other. Competitive sports serve as a civilized means of coexistence, offering a structured alternative to conflict and war. The rules governing sports become symbolic representations of civilization **(Fig. 1.5)**, embodying principles that facilitate harmonious interaction and competition on both individual and international levels.

When conducted effectively, sports have historically elevated the standards of nations to remarkable degrees. The contemporary media landscape is playing an unprecedented role in promoting sports, contributing to a significant surge in public interest. Participation in sports is widely acknowledged as a beneficial, accessible, and popular avenue for exercise and improved fitness. This surge in sports engagement has been fueled by increased school and community involvement, including coaching schemes at local centers. Additionally, the expansion of leisure time and improvements in healthy life expectancy have extended sports participation well into and beyond middle age.

While sports participation offers indisputable advantages, including enhanced physical fitness, cardiovascular performance, strength, speed, and improved response and reaction times, these benefits must be weighed against potential adverse effects. These drawbacks may encompass drawbacks in terms of time, financial investment, and competitive stress, particularly when performance falls short. More significantly, there is a looming risk of injury.

Undesirable elements such as hooliganism, professional fouls, incidents like gouging in rugby or elbow injuries in soccer, as well as broader issues

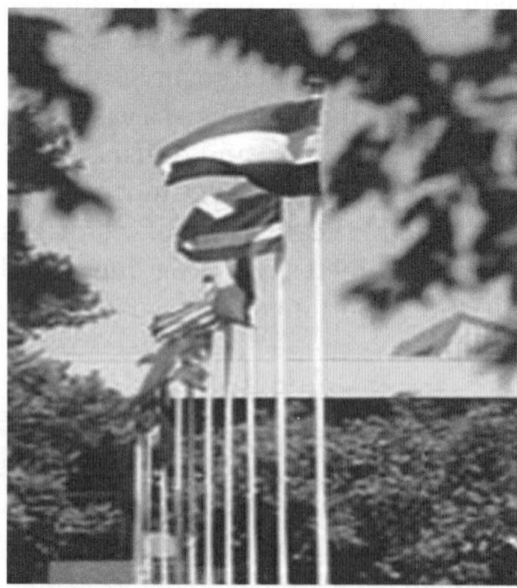

Fig. 1.5: Sports-mark of civilizations and harmony among different nations.

such as assault, bribery, drug abuse, racism, and political boycotts, represent unfortunate byproducts of contemporary sports. These challenges reflect a malaise within society and stand as a contradiction to the ideals of sportsmanship. Addressing these issues is crucial for safeguarding the integrity of sports and preserving the positive impact they can have on individuals and societies.

Sports serve as an enjoyable avenue for instilling lasting values and life lessons. They actively promote friendship and fair play while imparting essential qualities such as teamwork, discipline, respect, and patience. These skills are instrumental in nurturing children into compassionate individuals. Beyond physical fitness, sports play a pivotal role in preparing young people to confront challenges, fostering leadership skills that extend to community roles.

Crucially, sports teach humility in victory, emphasizing the genuine recognition of talent in others. The broader message is that, ultimately, we all depend on one another. The collective nature of sports encourages a sense of interconnectedness and mutual reliance. By engaging in sports, individuals not only develop their physical capabilities but also cultivate a rich tapestry of values that extend well beyond the playing field, contributing to their personal growth and positive engagement within their communities.

Vision

2 CHAPTER

Vision is the remarkable ability of the human body to perceive and interpret visual stimuli from the surrounding environment. It encompasses the intricate process by which the eyes capture images, transmit them to the brain, and translate them into meaningful information. This process, often taken for granted, is essential for spatial awareness, discrimination, and effective response to visual stimuli.

The process of vision begins with the eyes, which serve as the primary sensory organs for sight. Through a complex interplay of light, lenses, and receptors, the eyes capture incoming visual stimuli and convert them into electrical signals. These signals are then transmitted along the optic nerve to the brain, where they undergo interpretation, integration, and analysis **(Fig. 2.1)**.

The brain plays a central role in the process of vision, as it is responsible for fusing the images received from both eyes into a coherent three-dimensional representation of the environment. This integration enables individuals to perceive depth, distance, and spatial relationships accurately.

Vision involves more than just the physical act of seeing; it encompasses the ability to analyze, interpret, and respond to visual stimuli effectively. This cognitive aspect of vision enables individuals to make sense of their surroundings, recognize objects, and navigate their environment with ease.

Good vision is characterized by several key attributes, including spatial awareness, efficient discrimination, and the ability to sustain visual tasks without discomfort. It enables individuals to perform various visual tasks seamlessly throughout the day, regardless of the task or environmental conditions.

While vision is often considered a self-directed process, it can also be influenced by external factors such as lighting, environmental conditions, and individual preferences. Moreover, vision is not static; it can be refined and improved through practice, corrective measures such as spectacles or contact lenses, and refractive surgeries.

In summary, vision is a multifaceted process that involves the intricate interplay of the eyes, brain, and environment. It enables individuals to perceive, interpret, and respond to visual stimuli effectively, facilitating a deeper understanding of the world around them.

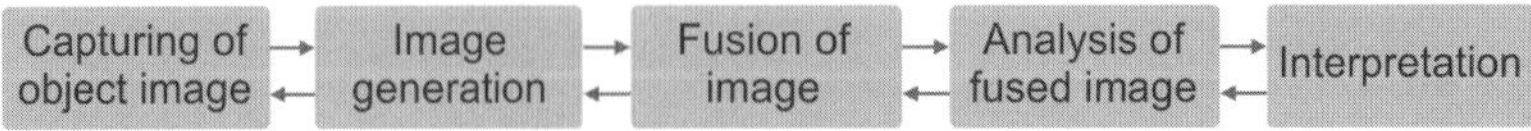

Fig. 2.1: Process of vision.

VISUAL SKILLS

Visual skills encompass a broad array of abilities that extend beyond mere visual acuity, such as 20/20 or 6/6 measurement. They encompass a variety of functions that enable individuals to perceive and interpret visual information effectively. Visual skills are shown in **Figure 2.2**.

Visual Acuity

Visual acuity is the time dependent measurement of retinal health and is specified by the date on which the eye examination took place. It is measured with the help of various eye test charts in a clinical environment. When measured on Snellen's test chart 20/20 or 6/6 signifies optimal visual acuity. However, it can be impaired by refractive errors, eye diseases like cataracts or glaucoma, and reduced contrast between objects and backgrounds.

Contrast sensitivity, vital for clear vision, diminishes in conditions like cataracts or retinal degeneration and with age, making it difficult to discern objects in low-contrast settings. Addressing contrast issues through glare control, optimal lighting, and appropriate lenses can significantly enhance visual acuity. Preserving visual acuity is essential for maximizing lifelong vision, promoting enjoyment of activities like sports, and potentially extending life expectancy through a healthier lifestyle. Therefore, maintaining good vision is pivotal for overall well-being.

An instant improvement in vision due to the use of correct filter or lens, will have a long-term effect on the preservation of visual acuity. Visual acuity needs to be preserved to maximize vision throughout life. This in turn will allow prolonged enjoyment of the sport and if a sport can be enjoyed, it will be

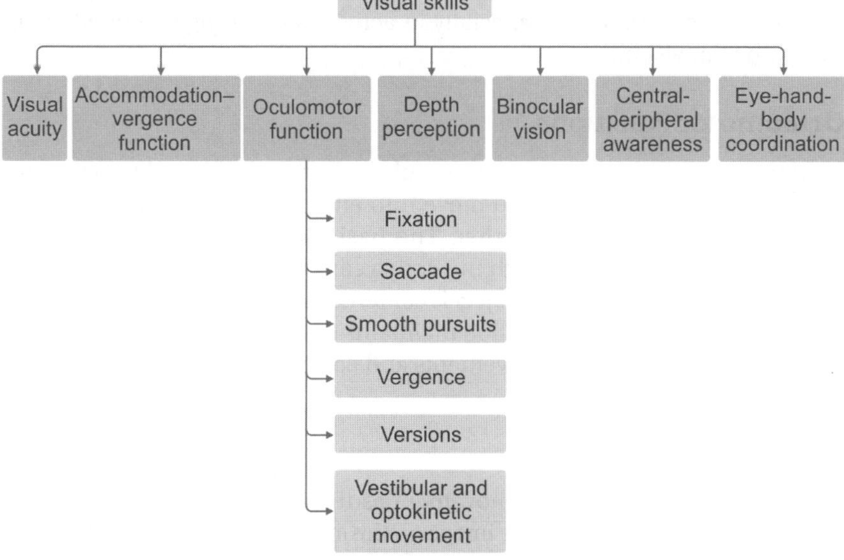

Fig. 2.2: Visual skills.

played for longer duration of life, which means the athletes maintain a healthy lifestyle, meaning potential to increase the life expectancy. This explains why vision is so much important for the life.

Accommodation–Vergence Function

Accommodation and vergence are essential functions of the visual system, enabling clear vision and binocular coordination. Accommodation is the eye's ability to adjust its focus to maintain clear images at varying distances, while vergence is the coordinated movement of both eyes to maintain binocular vision.

Accommodation involves the contraction of ciliary muscles, which changes the shape and focusing power of the lens. It allows clear vision at different distances. Accommodation function starts at the age of 3–4 months together with binocular vision, accommodation and appreciation of depth commence. From around 5 years of age to around 52 years of age, the amplitude of accommodation progressively decreases at a rate of approximately 0.30D/year.

Vergence, on the other hand, involves the simultaneous movement of both eyes to align their gaze on a single point. This movement is crucial for depth perception and spatial awareness. Vergence function directly controls muscle balance. The difficulties with muscle balance at distance or near are likely to affect visual performance directly. It may also increase the possibility of visual fatigue.

Both accommodation and vergence are closely linked and should work harmoniously for efficient vision. Changes in one function can affect the other, highlighting their interdependence. Proper assessment and management of accommodation and vergence issues are crucial for maintaining visual comfort and performance, especially in activities requiring sustained focus and binocular vision.

Oculomotor Functions

Oculomotor functions are neuromuscular controls developed to point the visual system on the target and move it to either follow a moving target or jump from one object to another. The basic skills are developed in the infancy and are refined through the early years. Clear vision occurs when a precisely focused image of an object is centered on the fovea and accurate eye movement or oculomotor function maintains the relationship.

The various types of eye movements and controls that help in clear vision are detailed below:

Fixation

Fixation is crucial during eye movement as the eye must remain still at the end of each saccade to focus the image on the fovea. This static phase requires coordination among all types of eye movements. Fixation ensures stable vision, enabling tasks like reading and focusing on objects.

Saccade

Saccades are rapid eye movements with a brief pause between them, allowing for a quick redirection of our line of sight to bring the point of interest to the fovea. Inaccuracy in saccades commonly occurs as a slight undershoot, where the movement falls short of the target, necessitating a corrective glide or a smaller second saccade. Less frequently, there may be an overshoot, where the eyes go beyond the intended target.

Smooth Pursuits

A pursuit eye movement tracks a moving object, matching the eye's velocity to that of the target. However, if the target moves too quickly, pursuits may become jerky. Factors like drugs, fatigue, stress, and anxiety can impair pursuit performance.

Vergence

Vergence is the simultaneous movement of both eyes in opposite directions to achieve or sustain binocular single vision. These movements occur when the eyes converge (move together) or diverge (move apart) when shifting focus between near and far objects. Vergence movements are slower compared to other eye movements and involve equal motion of both eyes in opposite directions. They are closely linked to accommodation of the eye.

Versions

Versions are eye movements that shift the direction of gaze towards a specific target, expanding the field of view to center the object of attention on the fovea. These movements, also known as conjugate eye movements, involve both eyes rotating through an equal angle in the same direction. Dextroversion refers to movement to the right, while levoversion indicates movement to the left. Versions can also occur vertically and torsionally.

Vestibular and Optokinetic Movements

The vestibular system greatly influences eye movements by providing sensory information about motion, equilibrium, and spatial orientation. This interaction is known as the vestibulo-ocular reflex, which stabilizes images on the retina during head movement. This is an orientation reflex, not requiring visual stimuli. Optokinetic reflexes, on the other hand, involve slow eye movements in response to moving images, allowing the eyes to track objects while the head remains still.

Depth Perception

Depth perception **(Fig. 2.3)**, a crucial aspect of healthy vision, relies on stereo vision, which enables us to judge relative distances and perceive objects in three-dimensional space. It occurs through the fusion of slightly disparate images captured by both eyes, allowing us to appreciate depth and spatial orientation. Stereopsis, a key aspect of binocular vision, facilitates this process by combining images from both eyes into a single coherent image. Fusion occurs when the brain is able to bring the two disparate images together and interpret them as one single image. There has to be fusion first before we can have depth perception.

Individuals with only one functioning eye often adapt to maintain reasonable depth perception for daily tasks, although higher-level skills may pose challenges. Depth perception is vital for everyday activities, such as gauging distances, determining approaching object speeds, and safely navigating environments.

Issues with depth perception may arise from various conditions, including blurred vision, strabismus, amblyopia, eye injuries, anisometropia, cranial nerve palsy, cataracts, macular degeneration, and anophthalmos. These conditions can affect the ability to perceive depth accurately and may impact daily activities like crossing streets safely.

Binocular Vision

Binocular vision involves the coordination of eye movements and the merging of sensory input from both eyes, enabling depth perception and detailed visual processing **(Fig. 2.4)**. The brain aligns and merges images from each eye, creating a unified three-dimensional picture.

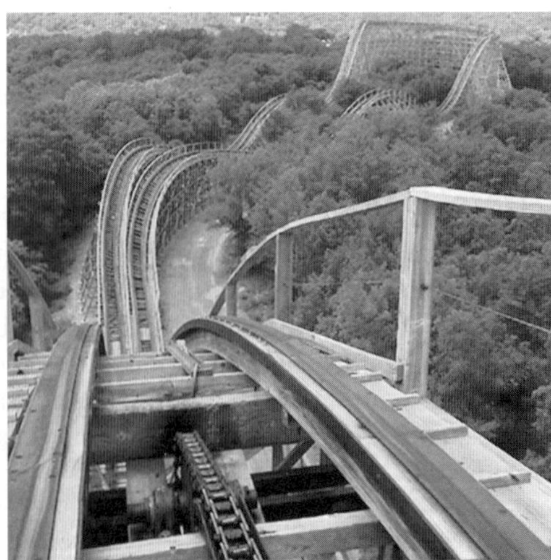

Fig. 2.3: Depth perception.

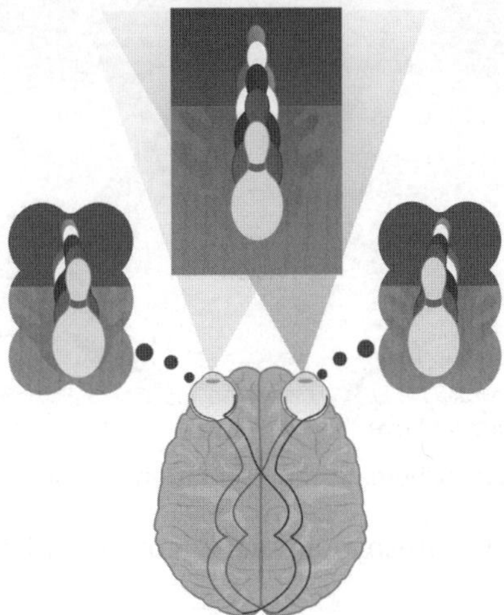

Fig. 2.4: Each eye captures its own view and the two separate images are sent on to the brain for processing. When the two images arrive simultaneously in the back of the brain, they are united into one picture.

Binocular vision offers several advantages:

- A broader field of vision, approximately 30 degrees wider than monocular vision.
- Improved visual acuity, typically half a line better on the Snellen's chart compared to either eye alone.
- Enhanced contrast perception by about 40% due to binocular summation of ocular images.

In binocular vision, one eye usually dominates visual consciousness and plays a primary role in seeing, while the other eye serves a supporting role. This dominant eye guides visual alignment, even when both eyes are open. The binocular projection center tends to be closer to the dominant eye.

Ocular dominance is a key concept in binocular vision, categorized into sensory, oculomotor, and directional dominance. Sensory dominance occurs when one eye is favored due to differences in image clarity, color, or brightness. Oculomotor dominance is evident when an eye better maintains central fixation despite fixation disparities. Directional dominance refers to which eye leads in fixating on a target, while the other eye follows at a slightly different angle, facilitating depth perception.

Eye dominance influences reading patterns. The right eye typically tracks from left to right, while the left eye naturally tracks from right to left. Individuals with left eye dominance may instinctively look at the right side of a page first and then move to the left, potentially causing challenges when reading languages that proceed from left to right, such as English.

Understanding ocular dominance is crucial for clinical assessments and treatments, such as prescribing prism lenses or implementing monovision correction techniques. In monovision, the dominant eye is corrected for distance vision, while the other eye is corrected for near vision, offering a

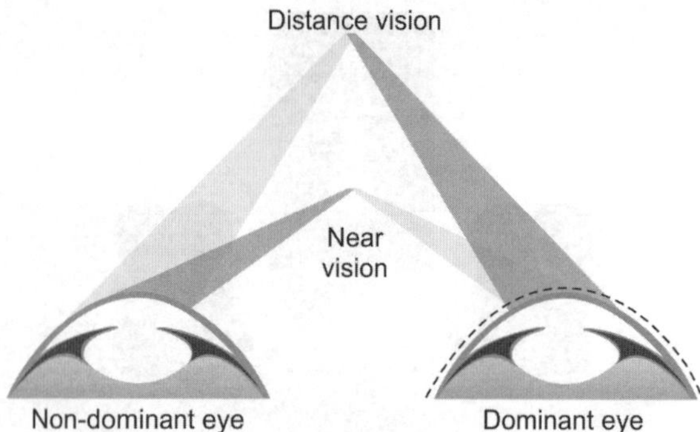

Fig. 2.5: Schematic representation of monovision.

successful approach for presbyopia management and refractive procedures **(Fig. 2.5)**.

Dominant eye suppression of a blurred image in the non-dominant eye may cause discomfort if the dominant eye's image is slightly blurred, even by just 0.25D, while a minor under-correction in the non-dominant eye may not be bothersome. Stable dominant eye characteristics are crucial for steady fixation on targets. Dominance conflicts can disrupt attention and comprehension, leading to binocular instability. Maintaining natural eye dominance is essential for visual stability and should not be disrupted.

Central-Peripheral Awareness

Central vision focuses on targets in the central portion of the visual field, while peripheral vision detects objects or actions outside the direct line of sight. Central-peripheral awareness enables simultaneous monitoring of both central and peripheral areas without turning the head, facilitating efficient reading and navigation.

Fixation, the shift from seeing everything to focusing on a specific object, occurs within about 3 degrees of the central visual field, where objects are seen in fine detail. Reduced peripheral vision in children may lead to distractions, decreased attention span, poor comprehension, and difficulties in tasks like reading and writing.

While central vision is prioritized due to its immediate threat detection capabilities, peripheral awareness is crucial for overall situational awareness. Peripheral vision can be compromised by conditions like glaucoma, strokes, head trauma, and stress, impacting movement detection and overall visual field.

Eye-Hand-Body Coordination

Eye-hand-body coordination encompasses the lightning-fast communication between the eyes, brain and body that allows us to effectively and efficiently use our hands and feet based on what we see. The process involves three steps and can be demonstrated by **Figure 2.6**.

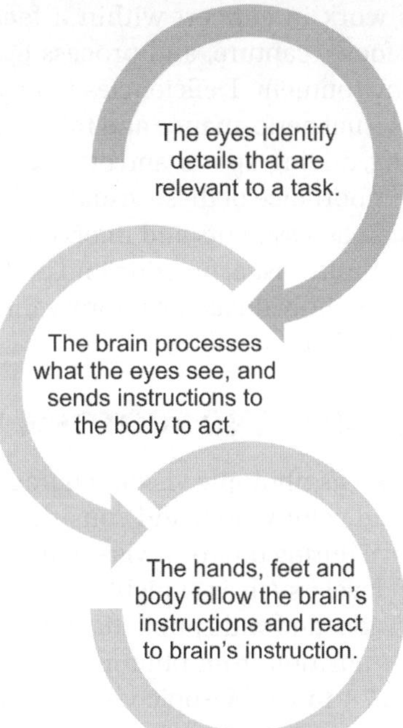

Fig. 2.6: Eye-hand-body coordination.

Eye-hand-body coordination is the rapid communication between the eyes, brain, and body that enables effective use of hands and feet-based on visual input. It involves the eyes leading and the body following, with good vision being fundamental. This coordination develops early in life and can be enhanced through exercises, requiring awareness of one's position and environment.

Developing eye-hand-body coordination involves various aspects:

- The vestibular system maintains balance and coordinates head and eye movements.
- Proprioception provides awareness of body movement and necessary force.
- Gross motor skills involve large muscle use for action.
- Fine motor skills utilize small muscles.
- Motor planning enables task completion without conscious effort.

Overall, eye-hand-body coordination demands integration of sensory and motor skills to perform tasks efficiently.

Additionally, the proprioceptive system encompasses the body's ability to sense its position, movement, and orientation in space. It plays a crucial role in coordinating visual information with other sensory inputs and motor responses, contributing to overall balance, coordination, and spatial awareness.

These visual skills work in concert within a feedback loop, allowing individuals to gather, focus, capture, and process light effectively to make sense of their visual environment. Deficiencies in any of these components can result in impaired visual performance and may manifest as difficulties in activities such as reading, driving, sports, and other visually demanding tasks.

Understanding the importance of these visual skills underscores the need for comprehensive vision assessments and interventions tailored to address individual needs and optimize visual function and performance. By nurturing and enhancing these skills, individuals can improve their overall visual health, comfort, and efficiency in daily activities.

PHOTOPIC, MESOPIC AND SCOTOPIC VISION

Daylight vision is termed as photopic vision, characterized by high acuity, low light sensitivity, good color vision, and constricted pupil aperture. Both rods and cones are active during photopic vision. In contrast, scotopic vision occurs in very low light levels, such as at night, showing high light sensitivity, poor acuity, no color vision, and wide pupil diameter.

Twilight marks the transition from photopic to mesopic and eventually scotopic vision **(Figs. 2.7A to C)**. Mesopic vision combines features of both photopic and scotopic vision, occurring in low but not entirely dark lighting conditions. In this range, both rods and cones are active, though rods dominate due to reduced light, leading to decreased color perception.

During twilight, some individuals may experience a shift towards low myopia, known as 'night myopia', due to reduced illumination. However, this is typically of minor significance. The transition between photopic and scotopic vision highlights the dynamic nature of visual adaptation to varying light levels.

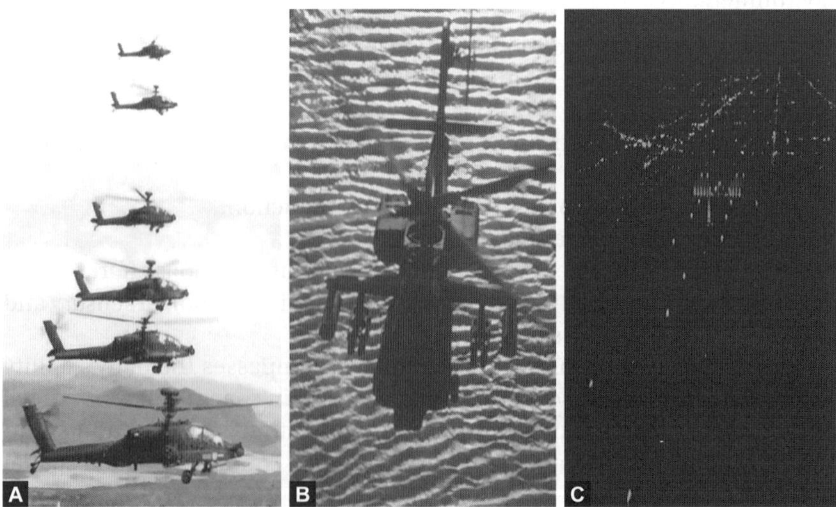

Figs. 2.7A to C: A. Photopic vision; B. Mesopic vision; C. Scotopic vision.

EFFECT OF HIGH ALTITUDE ON VISUAL PERFORMANCE

High altitude vision encompasses the visual changes and challenges encountered by individuals at high elevations. These changes result from environmental factors such as decreased atmospheric pressure, lower oxygen levels, increased UV radiation exposure, and temperature fluctuations. Common issues include eye redness reported by rigid gas permeable (RGP) lens wearers and slight vision reduction experienced by soft lens wearers. Post-LASIK patients may also undergo visual acuity fluctuations due to temporary myopic shifts.

Some common visual disturbances associated with high altitude vision include:

Reduced Visual Acuity

At high altitudes, individuals may experience fluctuations in visual acuity, which can affect their ability to see objects clearly, especially in varying light conditions.

Color Perception Changes

While color perception is generally unaffected, some individuals may notice alterations in color intensity or clarity due to the high-altitude environment.

Glare Sensitivity

Glare effects are more pronounced at high altitudes, particularly in snow-covered regions. The intense reflection of sunlight off snow can cause discomfort and reduce visual performance temporarily.

Dryness and Irritation

The low humidity levels prevalent at high altitudes can lead to dryness and irritation of the eyes, making them more prone to discomfort and redness.

Visual Distortions

Some individuals may experience visual distortions, such as halos or blurriness, especially during rapid ascents or changes in altitude. Symptoms such as headache, fatigue, dizziness, and dehydration also affect visual reaction speed.

Hypoxia-related Effects

Decreased atmospheric oxygen pressure at higher altitudes leads to hypoxia, which impacts vision. Prolonged hypoxia increases retinal blood flow, potentially resulting in intraretinal hemorrhage. However, studies suggest that these retinal changes are reversible with time and can be prevented by gradual ascent and supplemental oxygen use.

To mitigate the impact of high altitude on vision, individuals are advised to ascend gradually, stay well-hydrated, protect their eyes from UV radiation with sunglasses or goggles, and use artificial tears to alleviate dryness and irritation. Additionally, proper eye care and regular breaks during high-altitude activities can help alleviate discomfort and maintain visual comfort and clarity.

EFFECT OF AQUATIC ENVIRONMENT ON VISUAL PERFORMANCE

The underwater environment significantly affects visual performance due to several factors **(Fig. 2.8)**. Unlike in air, there is minimal refraction of light underwater because the refractive index of water and the cornea are similar, leaving the crystalline lens responsible for refraction. Consequently, objects appear blurred, larger, and closer underwater than they do in the air. Additionally, light loss and scattering occur as light reflects off particles in the water, creating a veil-like blinding effect that obscures vision. As depth increases, more light is filtered out by the water, leading to selective absorption of colors; red is lost first, followed by yellow, resulting in objects appearing blue-gray at extreme depths, hence the blue hue of the deep sea.

When prescribing contact lenses for water sports, certain guidelines should be followed. It is advisable to avoid prescribing rigid lenses due to the higher risk of loss associated with this type of lens in water. Larger, thicker, and low water content lenses offer greater stability and may be more suitable for shorter durations of sports activities.

EFFECT OF INDOOR ENVIRONMENT ON VISUAL PERFORMANCE

An athlete's sporting performance depends on numerous variables, with visual comfort during the event being crucial. Indoor sports present a different

Fig. 2.8: Underwater imaging is plagued by poor visibility conditions.

environment compared to outdoor sports, with factors like illumination level, glare, contrast, and visual contact with the exterior affecting visual performance. The overall quality of the indoor environment, including air quality, humidity, and temperature, can also influence visual performance. Attention to these environmental factors can enhance both physiological and psychological well-being, thereby improving an athlete's sporting performance.

In non-dynamic sports or indoor environments with low humidity and airflow, contact lens comfort may decrease, especially when the eyes are static. Concentration can lead to common issues like contact lens dehydration, often exacerbated by infrequent and incomplete blinking. Adjusting to these factors can significantly enhance an athlete's visual comfort and overall performance.

Visual Fatigue

Visual fatigue is a multifaceted condition characterized by episodic or persistent discomfort related to the subconscious process of vision. It occurs when the visual system is under strain due to the demands of a task and the degree of precision required to perform it. Also known as eye strain or asthenopia, visual fatigue refers to discomfort or tiredness in the eyes that typically occurs after prolonged periods of activities that require intense focus or concentration, such as reading, using a computer, or staring at a screen for extended periods.

Visual fatigue encompasses a spectrum of symptoms arising from excessive stress on the various components of the visual apparatus. These symptoms may include:

- Eye discomfort, such as burning, itching, or dryness
- Blurred or fluctuating vision
- Headaches, particularly in the temples or behind the eyes
- Sensitivity to light
- Difficulty maintaining focus or concentrating
- Eye redness or irritation.

The manifestation of visual fatigue hinges on three primary factors:

Nature of the Visual Task

The complexity and duration of the visual task significantly impact the onset and severity of visual fatigue. Tasks that require sustained focus or involve rapid changes in visual stimuli are more likely to induce fatigue.

Efficiency of the Visual System

The efficiency of the visual system, including factors like visual acuity, binocular vision, and depth perception, influences susceptibility to visual fatigue. Individuals with underlying vision problems or those who have not had adequate rest may experience heightened symptoms.

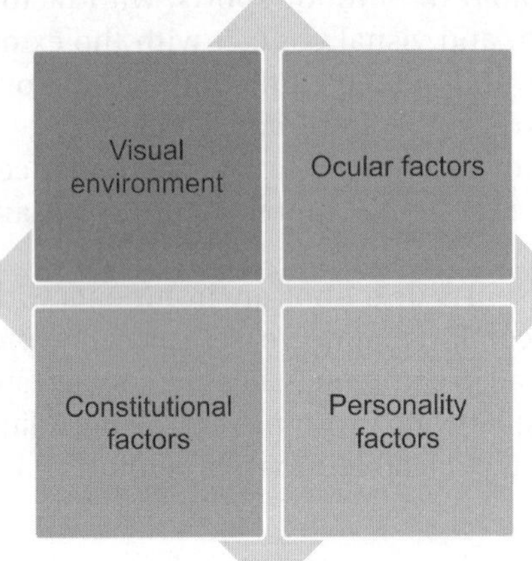

Fig. 2.9: Factors that are linked to vision fatigue.

Individual Capacity for Sustained Effort

Each person has a unique threshold for withstanding prolonged visual tasks. Factors such as age, overall health, and lifestyle can influence an individual's tolerance to visual strain.

Understanding visual fatigue requires consideration of multiple interrelated factors, which can be classified into four categories as shown in **Figure 2.9**.

Visual Environment

The visual environment for an individual encompasses all aspects of the surroundings that influence their visual perception and comfort. It includes both external and internal factors that impact how the individual perceives and interacts with their surroundings.

Lighting plays a critical role in the visual environment. It includes natural light from the sun as well as artificial lighting sources such as lamps, overhead lights, and electronic screens. The intensity, color, temperature, and distribution of light can affect visibility, comfort, and mood.

Glare refers to excessive brightness or reflection that can cause discomfort and reduce visibility. Glare sources may include direct sunlight, reflective surfaces, and poorly positioned light fixtures.

Contrast refers to the difference in brightness between objects or surfaces. High contrast can enhance visibility and clarity, while low contrast may make it difficult to distinguish details. Color also plays a role in the visual environment, influencing mood, perception, and visual appeal.

Visual stimuli encompass the objects, images, and patterns present in the environment. These stimuli can range from object size, object motion and colors to complex scenes and designs which can affect attention, perception, and cognitive processing.

Environmental conditions such as temperature, humidity, air quality, and noise levels can impact visual comfort and well-being. Extreme temperatures, poor air quality, and excessive noise can create discomfort and distraction, affecting visual performance and overall satisfaction with the environment.

The visual environment plays a pivotal role in inducing visual fatigue. It is essential to consider these factors in conjunction with other internal and external environmental elements.

Bright light, including sunlight and artificial glare, can trigger squinting as a protective mechanism to reduce the aperture of the pupil, shielding the eyes from potentially irritating or disturbing factors. Although squinting minimizes the impact of wide beam aberrations and also enhances visual input, prolonged squinting, achieved through muscle contraction, can lead to visual fatigue. The tension exerted on facial muscles during squinting can extend to other parts of the body, eventually resulting in general fatigue throughout the body. Dim light, on the other hand can contribute to visual fatigue through several mechanisms like increased effort to see, reduced contrast sensitivity, pupil size adaptation, increased sensitivity to glare, etc.

The environmental factors such as low contrast between details or high contrast between the task and its background can contribute to visual fatigue. Flickering from fluorescent lamps and the need for adequate ventilation also impact the visual environment and may exacerbate symptoms of fatigue.

Object size and motion can significantly impact visual fatigue due to the demands they impose on the visual system. Focusing on small objects for extended periods requires the eye muscles to maintain precise accommodation and convergence, leading to increased strain and fatigue. Tracking moving objects, such as scrolling text or dynamic images, demands continuous adjustments in eye movements and accommodation. Prolonged exposure to moving stimuli can lead to eye strain and fatigue, particularly if the motion is rapid or unpredictable.

High values of the parallax error also cause visual fatigue. Parallax error occurs when the apparent position or direction of an object appears to change depending on the observer's perspective. It commonly arises in situations where multiple objects are viewed from different vantage points, especially when one object is closer to the observer than another. Parallax results in disparity on the eye retinas. If the value of disparity is too high, oculomotor muscles are compelled to converge the eyes into unnatural positions, thus causing uncomfortable viewing situation.

Additionally, the overall satisfaction of an individual with their environment as a whole can influence the degree of visual fatigue experienced. Discomfort or dissatisfaction with environmental conditions can amplify the effects of visual strain.

Ocular Factors

Ocular factors contribute significantly to visual fatigue, with several conditions potentially causing strain and discomfort. These ocular factors include:

Uncorrected Refractive Errors

Refractive errors such as nearsightedness (myopia), farsightedness (hyperopia), and astigmatism can lead to visual fatigue when left uncorrected. Uncorrected refractive errors result in blurred vision, requiring the eyes to exert additional effort to focus properly.

Accommodative Insufficiency or Excess

Accommodative insufficiency occurs when the eye has difficulty adjusting its focus from distant to near objects, leading to eye strain during close-up tasks such as reading. Conversely, accommodative excess involves difficulty relaxing the focus when transitioning from near to distant objects, also contributing to eye strain.

Heterophoria

Heterophoria refers to a tendency for the eyes to deviate slightly from their normal alignment when not focusing. While mild heterophoria may not cause significant issues, sustained or excessive deviations can lead to eye strain and fatigue.

Convergence Difficulties

Convergence refers to the ability of the eyes to turn inward to maintain single binocular vision when focusing on nearby objects. Difficulties in convergence can result in double vision, eye discomfort, and visual fatigue, especially during prolonged close work. Breakdown of the accommodation and convergence relationship of the eye is the most common and frequent cause of the visual stress.

Fusional Inadequacy

Fusional inadequacy occurs when the eyes struggle to maintain binocular alignment under certain conditions, such as during extended periods of near work or when viewing objects at different distances. This can lead to symptoms of visual discomfort and fatigue.

Aniseikonia

Aniseikonia refers to a condition where the eyes perceive images of different sizes, leading to visual discomfort and strain, particularly during binocular viewing.

Uncorrected prescriptions or binocular instabilities contribute significantly to visual fatigue by disrupting the clarity and coordination of vision. When images are not properly focused on the retina, unclear signals are sent to the brain, prompting other ocular functions to compensate for the blurred image. The breakdown of the accommodation and convergence relationship is one of the most common causes of visual stress, as it disrupts the eyes' ability to maintain clear and comfortable vision, especially during sustained visual tasks.

Addressing ocular factors associated with visual fatigue often involves comprehensive eye examinations to identify and correct refractive errors, prescribe appropriate corrective lenses, and provide vision therapy or other interventions to improve accommodative and binocular function. By addressing underlying ocular issues, individuals can alleviate visual strain and enhance overall visual comfort and efficiency.

Constitutional Factors

Constitutional factors encompass both the physical and mental attributes of an individual. A breaking point is more likely to be reached in individuals with weaker constitutions compared to those who are robust. Symptoms tend to emerge more rapidly in those who are debilitated or in the process of recovering from an acute illness. Moreover, constitutional factors extend beyond the physical realm to encompass mental and emotional well-being. Insufficient sleep, heightened anxiety, and emotional strain are common manifestations of constitutional imbalances. These factors not only affect an individual's ability to cope with stress but also impact their overall quality of life and resilience in the face of challenges.

Personality Factors

Personality factors are also critical. Sometimes it's not what happens that matters but how you react to it that matters, which means it's not about the situation or the circumstance; it's about the personality of an individual. Personality factors indeed play a significant role in how individuals perceive and respond to various situations, including experiences of visual fatigue. Visual fatigue, often resulting from prolonged exposure to screens or intense visual tasks, can vary widely in its impact based on individual personality traits and coping mechanisms.

Individuals with resilient personalities tend to bounce back more easily from challenges, including visual fatigue. They may employ effective coping strategies such as taking regular breaks, practicing relaxation techniques, or adjusting their environment to reduce eye strain. In contrast, those with less adaptive coping styles may experience heightened distress and discomfort in response to visual fatigue, potentially exacerbating its effects. Optimistic individuals are more likely to maintain a positive outlook even in the face of visual fatigue. They may view it as a temporary inconvenience rather than a significant problem, which can help mitigate its impact on their overall well-being. Individuals who are adaptable and flexible in their approach to tasks and challenges may be better equipped to manage visual fatigue. Certain personality traits, such as neuroticism or perfectionism, can influence how individuals perceive and respond to visual fatigue. Those prone to perfectionism may push themselves to continue working despite experiencing discomfort, exacerbating their symptoms. On the other hand, individuals with a more laid-back attitude may prioritize self-care and recognize the importance of addressing visual fatigue promptly. In summary, personality factors significantly influence how individuals perceive, respond to, and cope with visual fatigue.

Visual fatigue is an often neglected in routine examination, but it has profound effect on the ability of an individual in highly visually demanding occupations like sports as it affects athlete performance adversely because of decreased quality of visual input that results in poor and slow decisions and reduces reaction time. Therefore, the diagnosis and management of visual fatigue is important. However, it is very complex because symptoms that are usually referred often seem to far from ocular origin. Secondly, in most cases distress is caused by such a small error that they easily escape detection unless they are looked for with extreme care. A holistic eye examination including the individual examination of all visual functions together with an assessment of the individual capabilities is required to determine whether the visual abilities match the visual requirement of the occupation. The treatment is not planned for the eye as an optical instrument only but is planned considering eye to be the integral part of the rest of the body, sharing with other organs in its constitutional variations and in the effects of the ills with which it may be afflicted.

Sports and Vision

3 CHAPTER

Sports represent a highly diverse array of occupations, each with its unique set of visual demands required to navigate effectively within its specific domain. Similar to any other profession, the visual requisites in sports exhibit a rich tapestry of diversity and complexity. Even within a particular sport, distinct positions may impose varying visual demands on athletes.

Understanding the different characteristics of sports, such as the control needed or the explosive nature of movements, underscores the inherent visual demands associated with athletic pursuits. The adage "You cannot hit it if you cannot see it!" or "You cannot catch it if you cannot see it!" succinctly captures the intuitive understanding of the pivotal role vision plays in sports.

In the fiercely competitive world of sports, athletes are in perpetual pursuit of that elusive factor that can provide them with a distinct advantage over their rivals. Research consistently supports the notion that "VISION" stands out as a critical element contributing significantly to an athlete's performance. In this context, vision is not merely about eyesight but encompasses the ability to perceive and process information swiftly and accurately, enabling athletes to make split-second decisions crucial to success.

As athletes continue pushing the boundaries of human performance, the recognition and enhancement of visual capabilities have become integral components of comprehensive training programs. The pursuit of excellence in sports now involves a holistic approach that includes not only physical conditioning but also the refinement and optimization of crucial visual skills.

In essence, the multifaceted nature of visual demands in sports underscores its importance as a decisive factor in achieving success. The athlete's ability to see, interprets, and respond to the dynamic challenges of their chosen sport plays a pivotal role in gaining a competitive edge. Therefore, the emphasis on refining visual acuity has become a strategic focus for athletes seeking to elevate their performance to new heights in the demanding and competitive world of sports.

In the realm of sports, a fundamental principle holds true: the eyes lead, and the body follows. Extensive research underscores the critical role that visual performance plays in shaping an individual's sporting development throughout their life. The relationship between vision and athletic potential is well-established, highlighting that any deficiency in visual performance can hinder an athlete's overall capabilities.

In the context of "sportvision," the term "vision" encompasses much more than the ability to read the bottom line of a text chart. It includes host of other visual facilities. It encompasses a spectrum of visual facilities that collectively contribute to an athlete's prowess.

Research in the field of sportvision over recent years has yielded intriguing findings that establish a clear link between sporting performance and visual capabilities. Studies consistently demonstrate that athletes and players at the elite level possess superior visual skills compared to the non-sporting population.

The incidence of eye dominance varies significantly across different sports. For example, in archery, 80% of athletes exhibit right-eye and right-hand dominance, while yachting tends to show a prevalence of left-eye dominance. Cricket, on the other hand, presents a more balanced distribution, with 50% right-eye dominance and 50% cross dominance. These findings suggest a potential predisposition of individuals with specific dominance to certain sports, or alternatively, a particular dominance configuration may develop over time within a specific sporting context.

A fascinating correlation emerges between the speed of eyes and the nature of fast-paced sports. In activities like downhill skiing and ice hockey, athletes develop eye speed to levels that can be considered almost superhuman. The speed of the eyes is a phenomenon intricately linked to the rapid movements required in these sports and is controlled by the speed of extraocular muscles.

The above findings underscore a conclusive connection between an athlete's sporting performance and their visual capabilities. There is a compelling suggestion that an individual's specific visual characteristics might serve as a decisive factor influencing their choice of a particular sport. Elite athletes consistently exhibit superior visual skills when compared to the general population, with advantages such as enhanced binocular vision, low phorias, improved stereopsis, and superior eye movement abilities.

■ PRIMARY VISUAL SKILLS IN SPORTS

The specific vision requirements of each individual sport need a combination of the two primary visual skills of aiming and anticipation. The proportion of one to another varies, from nearly all aiming, in sports like rifle shooting to nearly all anticipation in sports like tennis.

Let's delve deeper into the specific vision requirements and components of some of the sports.

Rifle Shooting

Aiming: Nearly all aiming is required in rifle shooting. This involves directing and maintaining steady, central visual attention on the target.

Vision skills: The shooter needs precise control over eye movements, especially during fixation, to align the sights accurately with the target.

Tennis

Anticipation: Tennis relies heavily on anticipation, where players need to predict the trajectory and speed of the incoming ball.

Vision skills: The ability to track the ball's movement and predict its path is crucial. This involves dynamic visual attention and quick decision-making.

Golf and Snooker

Aiming and anticipation: Both sports involve a balance between aiming and anticipation, with approximately 50:50 ratio.

Vision skills: Golfers and snooker players need to aim accurately, i.e., maintain steady visual attention on the target and anticipate factors like ball movement, trajectory, and environmental conditions.

Archery and Clay Pigeon

Aiming: Archery and clay pigeon are primarily an aiming sport where archers aim at a static target.

Vision skills: Precision in eye movements is crucial for fixating on the target, aligning the bow, and releasing the arrow accurately.

Football and Squash

Anticipation: Football and squash are predominantly anticipatory, requiring players to predict the movement of the ball, teammates, and opponents.

Vision skills: Players need to have excellent peripheral vision, quick decision-making abilities, and the capacity to anticipate the actions of multiple players simultaneously.

Cricket

Batting: Batting in cricket is predominantly anticipatory, involving predicting the bowler's delivery and reacting accordingly.

Bowling: Bowling, on the other hand, requires more aiming, with bowlers focusing on a specific target area.

Aiming is the ability to direct and maintain steady, central visual attention on the target. It involves correct positioning of the sights in relation to the location of the target. Aiming is achieved when the eyes fixate at an object. This is important as the eyes have to be static at the end of each saccade so that it can hold the image of interest on the fovea. Fixation is achieved through the combined involvement of all four eye movements, i.e., saccades, pursuits, vestibular ocular reflex and vergences. This is a well-integrated sensory-motor process where ocular muscles are in dynamic equilibrium.

There are four conditions that must be present for fixation to occur:
1. Good foveal function
2. Object to be fixated must have distinct contours
3. The object must have attention value
4. There must be sense of direction associated with foveal vision, which is likely to be absent in an eye which has abnormal retinal correspondence.

Absence of the above condition will discourage fixation and so it will reduce the time that is spent looking at the object. If the subject cannot maintain steady fixation, possible reasons could be:

- **Poor foveal function**, the fovea is the central part of the retina responsible for sharp central vision.
- **Indistinct contours of the object**; fixation is facilitated when the object to be fixed has clear and well-defined edges. The disrupting factors are poor lighting conditions, objects obscuring contours, the presence of visual clutter or distractions, etc.
- **Lack of attention value in the object makes fixation** more difficult, which may be because the object lacks attention holding or relevance, lack of interest or motivation in the task or distractions diverting attention from the target.
- **Absence of sense of direction in foveal vision, fixation** is influenced by the sense of direction associated with foveal vision. The disrupting factors are abnormal retinal correspondence affecting the perception of direction and disorders disrupting the neural pathways responsible for directional vision.
- **Ocular muscle imbalance**, an imbalance in the coordination of ocular muscles can affect fixation. The other factors that can affect ocular muscle balance are weakness or tightness in specific eye muscles and neurological conditions impacting muscle control, congenital nystagmus.
- **Vestibular dysfunction**, the vestibular ocular reflex contributes to fixation; dysfunction may disrupt this. Inner ear disorders affecting vestibular function and neurological issues impacting reflex coordination affect vestibular function.
- **Saccadic dysfunction, saccades** play a role in changing fixation points; dysfunction can lead to an unsteady gaze.
- **Cognitive and psychological** factors like anxiety or lack of concentration can impact fixation. Performance anxiety, stress, fatigue and drug effects affect fixation.

Improvement in fixation or aiming ability is often possible through appropriate environmental changes and functional vision training procedures. The basic skill is developed in infancy and refined through the early years. In sports, while aiming, generally there is an alignment. In the serve and volley game, the arm and the ball are relatively in alignment, which is halfway between true aiming and no aiming at all. In rifle shooting, the shooter has to align the front sight and the rear sight perfectly and consistently. There are four things in alignment before the shooter shoots—the aiming eye, the rear sight, the front sight, and the target. So it is a classic example of aiming for dominance. In golf, aiming is achieved by generalizing the direction of the target, assuming it to be through the center of the fairway, with peripheral awareness and a sideways stance to fix up the body and then hit the ball. In football, the ball is kicked by lining up the foot, the aiming eye, and the goal. In fencing, the tip of the foil and a target on the body of the opponent is aligned with the aiming eye.

Anticipation is the ability of an athlete to judge the speed and direction of the ball. It is the ability to block, hit, or avoid a rapidly moving object. The athlete anticipates the expected trajectory and the speed of the ball, decides a course of action, and then responds. If the athlete can anticipate quickly, he gets extra time to plan his response. The understanding, therefore, is that having good reflexes may not necessarily guarantee a successful, timely hit. Quick anticipation may make up for the physical limitations of reaction time. The ability to anticipate or "predict" an upcoming shot in tennis or the direction of a penalty kick in football allows players crucial time that they can dedicate to both getting to and preparing for an effective response. What makes the difference between a good player and a great player, apart from physical development, is the ability to anticipate.

Anticipation is very critical in elite sports, as the player has very limited time to:

- Judge the speed and direction of the ball
- Move and get in the right position for the return
- Decide where to hit the return shot and
- Prepare for and execute the stroke needed for the desired return.

The ability to anticipate is a function of depth perception. Depth perception is an important aspect of healthy binocular vision and a result of good stereovision. Stereovision is the ability to visually judge relative distances between objects and is a perceptual skill that aids accurate movement in three-dimensional space. The ability to anticipate is very much affected by a host of visual skills that are amenable to investigation, correction, and therapy.

Aiming is a precision skill that involves aligning the sights accurately with the target's location. The critical factors for successful aiming are focusing and convergence abilities. The dominant eye, which fixates on the target, plays a pivotal role in aiming, transmitting information to the brain milliseconds faster than the non-dominant eye. This dominant eye also guides the movement and fixation of the other eye, which aids in assessing distance and the spatial relationship of surrounding objects.

The significance of aiming, particularly in archery, is evident for strongly right-dominant athletes who can shoot without closing their non-dominant (left) eye. Keeping both eyes open in a right-dominant and right-hand dominant athlete maximizes acuity, contrast sensitivity, depth perception, and peripheral awareness during aiming, preventing fatigue in the eye muscles. Conversely, a left-dominant eye in a right-handed archer may require occlusion to prevent it from taking over.

While aiming, generally there is an alignment. When a team player hits, nothing is in alignment, but in a serve and volley game, the arm and the ball are relatively in alignment, which is halfway between true aiming and no aiming at all. Aiming is very important in fixed-target sports like rifle shooting. Difficulties in aiming are also seen when there is no fixed target, like in golf. In golf, aiming is achieved by generalizing the direction of the target, assuming it to be through the center of the fairway, with peripheral awareness and a sideways stance to fix up the body and then hit the ball. In football, the ball is kicked by lining up the foot, the aiming eye, and the goal. In fencing, similarly, the tip of the foil and a target are on the body of the opponent.

Anticipation, involving the prediction of actions such as the trajectory of a tennis ball or the spin of a cricket ball, plays a crucial role in improving response time. It can compensate for physical limitations in reaction time and is influenced by various visual skills, including eye movements, visual acuity, contrast sensitivity, accommodation facility, glare recovery, and eye-hand coordination. These visual skills are subject to investigation, correction, and therapeutic interventions.

The ability to anticipate relies heavily on the rapid interpretation of visual cues such as ball spin, gaze direction, bat movement, body positioning, wind direction, racket angle, hand grip, and more. Physiologically, the human visual system's limitations stem from the speed at which sensory input is transmitted—how quickly the image of the ball travels from the eyes to the brain. Physical strength also plays a role to some extent. Beyond physical prowess, what distinguishes a great player from a good one is their adeptness at anticipation.

Anticipation is intricately connected to depth perception, a crucial element of normal binocular vision. A healthy binocular vision, achieved through proficient stereo vision, facilitates precise judgment of relative distances between objects, enhancing spatial awareness in three-dimensional space. The loss of binocular depth perception significantly hampers participation in sports, underscoring the pivotal role of establishing binocular vision early in life for the development of stereopsis.

The absence of binocular depth perception deprives individuals of engaging fully in various sports. It is essential to recognize that the ability to perceive depth is not innate and requires the early establishment of binocular vision for the proper development of stereopsis. The lack of binocular vision represents a significant visual disability that merits heightened attention.

The consequences of losing binocular vision extend beyond sports, impacting overall quality of life and limiting life choices. Athletes, in particular, should be mindful of these implications. Raising awareness about the importance of maintaining and developing binocular vision can lead to early intervention and appropriate corrective measures.

In summary, the intricate relationship between anticipation, depth perception, and binocular vision underscores the significance of visual skills in sports. The loss of binocular vision not only affects athletic performance but also has broader implications for an individual's daily life. Recognizing and addressing this issue can contribute to a more comprehensive understanding of visual health and its impact on overall well-being.

FACTORS AFFECTING AIMING AND ANTICIPATION

Aiming and anticipation in sports can be influenced in more than one way by several visual skills.

Visual Acuity

Visual acuity plays a pivotal role in an athlete's ability to discern crucial visual cues such as a bowler's hand grip or the trajectory of a ball in flight, allowing them to effectively focus on the target. The fundamental principle is that clear visibility of the target is essential for accurate fixation; if the target is not seen clearly, fixation becomes challenging. Excellent visual acuity implies sharp foveal vision, a critical factor in sports aiming.

The contrast between the object and its background significantly influences an athlete's aiming ability. Poor contrast, often exacerbated by adverse weather conditions such as rain, sleet, haze, air pollution, darkness, or various lighting conditions in a stadium, can impede an athlete's contrast sensitivity. Additionally, factors like glare from bright sun or stadium lights, as well as overcast conditions, create a veiling effect that further impacts contrast sensitivity.

Contrast sensitivity is also influenced by the velocity of the moving object. High-speed movements, characteristic of many sports, demand optimal contrast for athletes to quickly discern and lock onto their targets. Adverse conditions or inadequate contrast can hinder an athlete's ability to pick up fast-moving targets efficiently.

Accommodation–Vergence Function

The accommodation function plays a crucial role in an athlete's ability to swiftly shift focus from one object to another. Any compromise in this function can result in premature eye fatigue, leading to delays in the aiming process. The athlete's ability to quickly and accurately adjust focus is fundamental to maintaining optimal performance.

Vergence, the ability to seamlessly fuse two images from both eyes into a single image during changes in focus (divergence from near to far and convergence from far to near), is vital for visual coordination. The eyes collaborate to sustain this fusion across all directions of gaze. Any deficiency in vergence can lead to double vision, hindering an athlete's anticipation, reaction time, and overall performance.

The speed and accuracy of the eye's converging ability are particularly critical in sports that involve tracking fast-moving targets, such as following a small and swiftly moving puck in ice hockey. The convergence skill enables the athlete to precisely focus on the target, facilitating a more effective and timely response.

Oculomotor Function

The oculomotor function of the eye controls the position and movement of the eyes to focus the image of the visual target on corresponding areas of the retinas of the two eyes. Eye movements are also controlled and executed by the extraocular muscles. Fixation is an important consideration during aiming because the eye has to be static at the end of each saccade as it holds the image of the object on the fovea. Fixation needs the combined involvement of all types of eye movements. This is a well-integrated sensory-motor process where the muscles are in dynamic equilibrium.

In sports, the ability to maintain fixation on rapidly moving objects is a critical aspect of allowing the visual processing of crucial information. It also enables changing fixation from one point to another rapidly and accurately in dynamic sports and is critical to maintaining steady fixation in non-dynamic sports like target shooting. The accuracy of the ocular alignment of the two eyes on a given target depends upon the amount of innervations exerted by each of the six extraocular muscles in each eye that provide precise anticipation by depth perception for successful sporting performance. The speed and precision of the extraocular muscles are very important for aiming and anticipation in sports. However, the need for it can vary from one sport to another.

Geraint Griffiths has categorically mentioned in his paper *'Eye speed, motility and athletic potential'* that fast eyes are associated with fast sports. In modern sports like downhill skiers traveling at a speed of 80 mph and ice-hockey player trying to hit a small dangerous puck, develops the eye speed to almost superhuman levels. Whether the game is fast moving like ice-hockey or slower and more thoughtful like curling, it is likely to be an advantage if the athlete has good oculomotor control and cognitive ability.

The speed and precision of extraocular muscles are paramount for aiming and anticipation in sports, although the extent of this requirement may vary across different sports.

Depth Perception

The ability to anticipate in sports is intricately tied to depth perception—a crucial aspect of healthy binocular vision and a byproduct of effective stereo vision. Depth perception involves spatial judgment, allowing athletes to assess the distance between themselves, the ball, teammates, opponents, boundary lines, and other objects on the field.

In football, depth perception proves to be of utmost importance for players in various positions. Efficient and accurate perception of the ball's spatial position, coupled with a keen understanding of its speed and trajectory, directly influences the timing of eye, hand, body, and foot responses. A notable example of the significance of depth perception in football is evident when a player needs to skillfully pass the ball beyond the reach of defenders and into the goalpost. This skill requires a precise understanding of the spatial relationships in the field.

The role of depth perception extends to anticipating the ball in flight, prompting players to adjust their positions accordingly to receive it. This dynamic process showcases how depth perception in football is not only about reacting to the current state of play but also involves anticipating future scenarios. The ability to accurately gauge distances, speeds, and trajectories enhances a player's strategic decision-making and execution on the field.

Binocular Vision

Binocular vision is a critical aspect for athletes as it enables the perception of depth, significantly influencing their ability to anticipate movements effectively. The appreciation of three-dimensional spaces is fully realized through binocular vision, making it a key factor in athletes' spatial awareness. Loss of binocular vision represents a serious visual disability that compromises stereopsis—the ability to perceive depth accurately—and subsequently hampers sporting performance.

In well-developed binocular vision, the dominant eye takes the lead in fixating at the target. This is particularly crucial in shooting sports, where the alignment of the dominant eye, hand, foresight of the gun, and the target determines accuracy. Strongly right-dominant shooters, e.g., can often shoot without occluding their left eye, maximizing visual acuity and peripheral awareness while preventing fatigue in the eye muscles.

The benefits of binocular vision extend beyond mere depth perception; it plays a pivotal role in enhancing precision and coordination in various sports. In shooting, the alignment facilitated by binocular vision not only aids accuracy but also contributes to overall visual comfort and stamina. Binocular vision is indispensable for athletes, providing them with the ability to perceive depth accurately and enhancing their anticipation skills. The loss of binocular vision poses a significant challenge in sports.

Central-Peripheral Awareness

The positioning of sights in relation to the target and the athlete's spatial orientation within the sports environment significantly influences aiming ability. When the athlete identifies a target, fixation typically occurs at the central portion of their visual field. Peripheral vision, on the other hand, serves to gather information from the sides without necessitating head movement. A fundamental principle in sports is to "keep the head as still as possible and minimize eye movement."

In activities such as boxing and motor racing, maintaining central peripheral awareness is not only crucial for performance but can also be a matter of life and death. This awareness, involving both central and peripheral vision, plays a pivotal role in aiming and anticipation. In tennis, for instance, where aiming is part of the game, peripheral awareness informs the athlete about the positions of opponents and the ball's trajectory, guiding their overall strategy on the court.

In hockey, players must constantly maintain spatial awareness through peripheral vision to anticipate the movements of teammates and opponents. This awareness is instrumental in predicting the speed and direction of the ball, enabling players to position themselves effectively and aim their sticks to make precise contact with the ball.

The interplay between central and peripheral vision is a critical aspect of aiming and anticipation in various sports. Athletes who manage the balance between central fixation and peripheral awareness enhance their overall performance by making informed decisions and executing precise actions based on their surroundings.

The integration of central and peripheral vision is vital for athletes in aiming and anticipation. It not only improves their spatial awareness within the sports environment but also influences their ability to make well-informed decisions and execute actions accurately, contributing to success in their respective sports.

Visual Clues

Visual clues play a pivotal role in shaping the anticipation ability of athletes, where the speed and accuracy of anticipation are closely tied to the swift interpretation of these cues. The adeptness in detecting advanced clues that foreshadow an opponent's response has the potential to elevate an athlete to a superior and advantageous level.

The athlete's ability to anticipate is intricately linked to the rapid processing of visual cues such as the spin of the ball, direction of gaze, speed and trajectory of the bat, body movements, wind direction, speed of approach, angle of the racket, hand grip, and more. In cricket, for example, a batsman focuses on the bowler's torso during the approach and shifts their gaze to the bowler's hand just before the ball is delivered. This process involves perceiving multiple visual cues, including the bowler's action, arm swing speed, body turns, and shoulder movements.

The batsman's anticipation hinges on accurately interpreting these visual clues to estimate the speed, line, and length of the incoming ball. Armed with this information, the batsman aligns their bat with the anticipated path of the ball, completing the aiming process and preparing for an effective shot.

The ability to anticipate in sports is heavily dependent on the athlete's capacity to rapidly and accurately process a multitude of visual cues. Success in anticipating opponent actions or predicting the trajectory of a moving object is a result of the athlete's keen visual acuity and interpretation skills, ultimately influencing the success of their aiming and response strategies in the game.

Prior Knowledge

Prior knowledge, derived from understanding how a specific opponent plays, serves as a valuable asset in hastening the anticipation of the speed and direction of the ball. This strategic advantage is the reason why many elite-level athletes diligently gather information about their opponents before a competition. This pre-existing knowledge allows athletes to make quicker and more accurate decisions during gameplay, enhancing their overall performance by anticipating and responding to the opponent's actions with greater efficiency.

Glare Recovery

Glare is a visual phenomenon that occurs when external light scatters within the eye, creating a hazy veil over the retinal surface. This effect diminishes the contrast of the retinal image, impacting both aiming and anticipation abilities. The reduction in contrast caused by glare can hinder an athlete's capacity to perceive visual cues accurately, potentially affecting their performance in tasks that require precise aiming and swift anticipation of dynamic movements.

In the process of binocular vision, the dominant eye takes the lead in fixating, followed by the non-dominant eye a few milliseconds later. The non-dominant eye gathers information to aid in determining distance and the spatial relationship of objects surrounding the point of focus. The ability to anticipate effectively relies heavily on the rapid interpretation of visual clues, requiring active accommodation, good vergence facility, visual acuity, contrast sensitivity, and binocular coordination. These aspects are assessable through diagnostic tests, providing opportunities for correction and improvement.

Physiologically, the human visual system is constrained by the speed at which sensory input is transmitted—how swiftly the image of the ball moves from the eyes to the brain. Additionally, the physical strength of the player plays a role in visual performance.

Aiming and anticipation are not exclusive to sports; they are inherent in daily activities from infancy. Children begin to use aiming as they become visually aware, reaching for objects in line with their aiming eye. Any issues with eye dominance can disrupt this process, affecting their ability to accurately perceive object locations in space.

As children start to walk and explore their surroundings, judging the position of objects becomes crucial for safety. Misjudgments can lead to collisions with sharp edges or obstacles, impacting mobility and confidence. Similarly, in sports, poor visual judgment inhibits performance and physical development.

In summary, aiming and anticipation are fundamental visual skills applicable across all sports and daily activities. Subtle changes in their efficiency can be frustrating for athletes, underscoring the importance of assessing and addressing visual skills for optimal performance and overall well-being.

Visual Demands in Sports

4 CHAPTER

Sports are highly visually demanding occupations. Athletes and players continuously take in visual inputs regarding the ball, other players and the surroundings, process the information to react, respond by moving hands, feet and body and finally complete visual task either by catching ball, hitting or throwing ball, kicking or punching the opponent. In the process, every facet of visual system plays is involved.

Athletes and players need sharp central vision to detect subtle movements, details, or changes in the environment. This is vital in sports like shooting, archery, and even activities like rock climbing.

Athletes need to maintain intense focus for extended periods. Visual concentration is required to block out distractions and stay attuned to the game or competition. This is essential in sports like gymnastics and figure skating.

Judging distances and depths accurately is essential in sports. Athletes need to assess the position of objects in their environment to make quick and accurate decisions. This skill is crucial in sports like golf, archery, and soccer.

Being aware of what's happening in the periphery is important in team sports. Athletes must be able to monitor the entire playing field or court while focusing on specific tasks. This is particularly important in sports like football and basketball.

Many sports require precise hand-eye coordination. Athletes need to accurately track moving objects, such as a ball or opponent, and coordinate their movements accordingly. This is crucial in sports like tennis, baseball, and basketball.

Sports often require split-second decision-making and rapid reactions. Athletes need to process visual information quickly and respond accordingly. This is evident in sports such as boxing, fencing, and hockey.

Athletes must predict the path of the object and position themselves accordingly. Following the trajectory of a fast-moving object, such as a ball or puck, is crucial in sports like cricket, baseball, and hockey.

Recognizing patterns and anticipating opponents' moves is crucial in strategic sports like chess, as well as in team sports where players need to understand the patterns of play.

Every facet of visual system is involved in the visual process. Understanding the implications of each facet is critical to develop a sport-specific visual profile for a specific sport and then identify the visual skill weaknesses for remediation and enhancement therapy. **Figure 4.1** shows the different facets of vision that are critical to understand to establish a comprehensive sport-

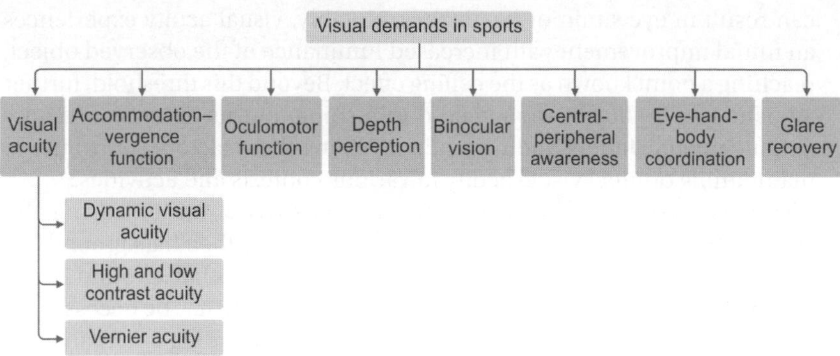

Fig. 4.1: Different facets of visual skills.

specific visual profile, targeted remediation and enhancement therapies to address specific weaknesses.

VISUAL ACUITY

Visual acuity is the spatial resolving capacity of the visual system, which affects aiming ability of the athletes. It is most commonly measured statically, and is therefore, also referred to as Static Visual Acuity (SVA). Visual acuity of an individual person depends upon host of factors which can be grouped under physical and physiological factors. Physical factors may be said to include those factors that directly or indirectly affect light and light transmission and thus influence the retinal image. Physiological factors are linked to an individual person. A broad level discussion on all factors can be done on several heads as shown in **Figure 4.2**.

- The object size and the object distance are the foremost important factor that determines the visual acuity of an individual. The physical size of the object and its distance from the eye determines the visual angle. The objects situated closer create larger visual angles compared to those at a greater distance. Similarly larger objects create larger visual angle. Therefore, the combination of object size and distance determines the clarity and detail with which an individual can perceive visual stimuli.
- The ability to perceive fine details is intricately linked to the intensity of illumination falling on the observed object. While the eye can detect faint sources and movements in comparatively low light conditions, recognizing intricate details necessitates sufficient illumination. Engaging in tasks that demand precision, such as reading or fine work, in inadequate lighting

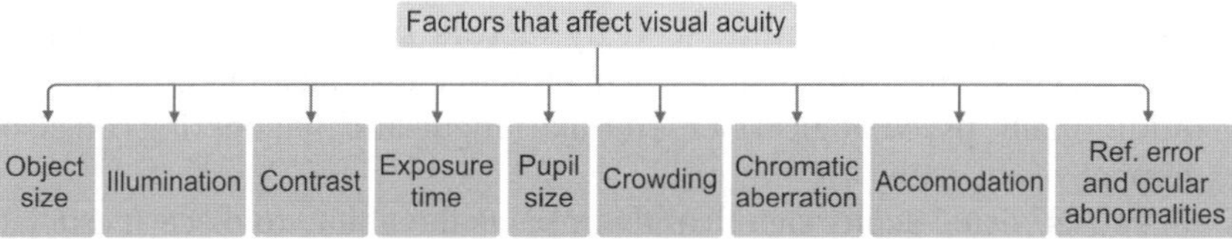

Fig. 4.2: Factors that affect visual acuity.

can result in eye strain or headaches. Notably, visual acuity experiences an initial improvement with increased luminance of the observed object, reaching a point known as the ceiling effect. Beyond this threshold, further adjustments in illumination yield diminishing returns in terms of acuity enhancement. Understanding and optimizing these factors contribute to maintaining optimal visual acuity in various contexts and activities.

- Vision is intricately linked to contrast sensitivity, underscoring the significance of clear distinctions between objects and their backgrounds. In situations where the contrast between an object and its background is low, compensatory measures, such as enlarging the object, may be necessary to achieve comparable levels of visual acuity. Understanding and managing contrast in the visual environment are key elements in optimizing visual acuity for various visual tasks and activities.
- The impact of exposure time on an individual's visual acuity is a subject with limited available evidence. However, it holds practical significance, particularly in the context of dynamic visual acuity, where either the object under observation, the observer, or both are in motion. Generally accepted is the notion that dynamic visual acuity tends to decrease when the exposure time or duration of observing an object is shorter.
- The size of the pupil plays a crucial role in determining visual acuity. A larger pupil allows more light to stimulate the retina, reducing diffraction, but it can be impacted by aberrations in the eye, affecting resolution. Conversely, a smaller pupil minimizes optical aberrations but limits resolution due to diffraction. Optimal visual acuity is often achieved with a mid-size pupil, typically ranging from 3 mm to 5 mm, striking a balance between diffraction and aberration limits.
- The interaction between two closely positioned objects can diminish visual acuity. This phenomenon, known as crowding, is frequently observed in individuals with amblyopia or severe maculopathy. Crowding imposes a fundamental constraint on conscious visual perception and hinders object recognition across the entire visual field.
- Using monochromatic light rather than white light is expected to yield a clearer image by eliminating the impact of chromatic aberrations.
- Form sense, predominantly governed by cones, is most acute at the fovea due to a higher concentration of cones, which diminishes rapidly towards the periphery. In the peripheral retina, cone sensitivity decreases, while rod sensitivity increases.
- Accommodation is crucial for achieving spatial resolution at different distances from the eye. A young emmetrope with an intact accommodative reflex can effectively perform visual tasks that involve depth scanning.
- Visual acuity may be influenced by factors such as refractive error, corneal curvature abnormalities, ocular media opacities, and axial length. Additionally, psychological elements like fatigue and malingering can also impact visual acuity.

In sports, visual acuity significantly impacts the ability to discern crucial visual cues, such as a bowler's hand grip or the trajectory of a ball in the air, and to fixate on the target. The fundamental principle is that clear visibility of the target enables effective fixation; conversely, if one is not looking directly at something, visibility is compromised. Good visual acuity, indicative of strong foveal vision, is particularly vital for precise aiming in sports.

In the sporting context, visual acuity is influenced by various factors, including:
- Target size and distance.
- Speed of the target.
- Speed of the athlete.
- Contrast of the target against its background.
- Color of the target and background.
- Ambient light level.
- Position of the luminaries.
- Precipitation and wind speed.
- Reflectivity of the playing surface and surroundings.
- Environmental distractions like rain, mist, fog, etc.

DYNAMIC VISUAL ACUITY

In the realm of sports, events are predominantly characterized by motion, involving either the athlete or the object in motion. This raises the argument that static visual acuity alone does not provide an accurate representation of visual acuity demands. To truly assess visual acuity, it is crucial to determine the Dynamic Visual Acuity (DVA) threshold. Dynamic visual acuity is defined as the ability to resolve details when there is relative movement between the observer and the test object.

The measure of visual acuity during relative motion between the object and the observer is termed as Dynamic Visual Acuity (DVA). Given the dynamic nature of most sports, DVA emerges as a potentially important variable in sports performance. Notably, there exists a modest correlation between Static and Dynamic Visual Acuity, with DVA showing a significant decrease as target velocity increases.

However, the measurement of dynamic visual acuity is not commonly incorporated into routine optometric examinations. While various research groups have endeavored to develop suitable tests for dynamic visual acuity, standardization remains limited. Nevertheless, there is a consensus that DVA is influenced by several factors:
- Poor static visual acuity makes it unlikely for dynamic visual acuity (DVA) to be satisfactory, and significant individual differences in DVA are noted among subjects with similar static visual acuity.
- DVA is influenced by learning, with practice enhancing DVA. Athletes engaged in dynamic sports often exhibit superior dynamic visual acuity.
- Fixation accuracy on a moving object involves the coordinated efforts of saccades, pursuits, vestibular ocular reflexes, and vergences to maintain a steady image on the fovea.
- Deterioration in DVA is observed with reduced contrast between the stimulus and its background, impacting static acuity.

- Dynamic visual acuity experiences a notable decline with increased target velocity during tracking movements.
- Males tend to have slightly higher dynamic visual acuity than females.
- Dynamic visual acuity deteriorates more rapidly with age compared to static visual acuity.
- Athletes in dynamic sports may develop enhanced dynamic visual acuity through consistent practice.
- Deficits in static visual acuity can hinder the perception of small objects or subtle facial expressions, while deficits in dynamic visual acuity affect timing, distance judgment, and the detailed observation of objects, such as discerning the spin of a ball.

Dynamic visual acuity (DVA) tests are designed to minimize variables by restricting either the target's or the subject's motion. When limiting target motion, subjects are encouraged to move their heads at a specific frequency, although precise measurement of this movement may be challenging. Alternatively, restricting target motion offers better control and monitoring possibilities.

It is important to note that DVA is linked to the efficiency of the entire visual system, with the oculomotor system playing a crucial role. Various eye movements contribute to this process. Smooth pursuit eye movements ensure the continuous foveation of the target during tracking. Saccadic catch-up, employed alongside the pursuit system, helps maintain foveation of the target. The vestibular ocular reflex, working in conjunction with saccades and pursuit eye movements, compensates for head, body, and external movements to preserve the retinal image. Clear vision is achieved when a precisely focused image of the object of regard is centered on the fovea, and accurate oculomotor skills maintain this relationship.

Dynamic visual acuity is intricately connected to the efficiency of the entire oculomotor system, where eye movements play a pivotal role. The eyes can accurately follow a target in motion up to a maximum velocity of approximately 40 degrees per second. Smooth pursuit eye movements ensure the ongoing foveation of the target during tracking, but beyond angular velocities of 40 degrees per second, accurate tracking becomes challenging.

Saccadic catch-up, working in conjunction with the pursuit system, is employed to maintain the foveation of the target. Saccades, characterized by ballistic movements, can be used to foveate intervals of a target trajectory, even at angular velocities reaching up to 1000 degrees per second.

Additionally, the vestibular ocular reflex collaborates with saccades and pursuit eye movements to compensate for head, body, and external movements. This reflex ensures the maintenance of a stable retinal image despite changes in the external environment.

HIGH AND LOW CONTRAST ACUITY

Sports take place in dynamic environmental conditions that impact visual performance by influencing contrast levels. Factors such as rain, sleet, haze, air pollution, indoor lighting, darkness, stadium lights, glare, bright sun, and overcast conditions all contribute to variations in contrast between the target and its background, consequently affecting visual performance.

Contrast sensitivity, as demonstrated by several studies, offers valuable insights into functional or real-world vision that may not be fully captured by a visual acuity test alone. Therefore, combining low-contrast acuity with high-contrast visual acuity provides clinicians with a more comprehensive understanding of an individual's actual visual functioning in real-world scenarios.

In various clinical scenarios, contrast sensitivity can be compromised even when visual acuity remains normal. Conditions such as refractive surgery, capsular opacification of lenses, oxidative changes due to heavy smoking, multiple sclerosis, and diabetes without significant retinopathy, cataract, age-related maculopathy, or corneal edema can lead to a reduction in contrast sensitivity.

In the context of sports, the dynamic and ever-changing environment poses challenges to discriminating objects, creating potential inaccuracies in the information processed by the brain. The velocity of object movement also adversely affects contrast sensitivity, indicating that high-speed scenarios demand higher levels of visual skills. Deficits in contrast sensitivity can impact an athlete's ability to pick up visual cues on the field, causing delays in reacting to a tennis ball or negotiating snow undulations while skiing. For instance, tracking a white ball against a light blue sky presents a low-contrast environment, underscoring the significant impact of contrast sensitivity on athletic performance.

The use of low-contrast charts proves to be more informative in assessing these scenarios. Athletes quickly recognize the relevance of measuring vision at low contrast, as it reflects real-life conditions such as poor lighting, fading sun, mist, rain, and dirty kit. Performance deficits at low contrast can be significant, even when high-contrast vision is reasonably good. Subtle visual deficiencies may not be apparent at high contrast, particularly under favorable lighting conditions. Disproportionate worsening of visual acuity at low contrast is usually indicative of an issue with the visual system, emphasizing the importance of low-contrast acuity in relation to real-life sports conditions.

VERNIER ACUITY

Vernier acuity serves as an alternative method for gauging potential vision. It pertains to the accuracy with which an individual can assess the alignment of targets, such as determining whether two spots are vertically aligned. Vernier acuity essentially involves the "recognition of relative position". During the test, the subject is prompted to evaluate the offset between two parallel lines, using both eyes and each eye individually. The test employs targets with progressively decreasing displacements until the subject can no longer differentiate the displacement. Vernier acuity for a subject is defined as the smallest visible offset between stimuli that can be detected. The precision of observations in vernier acuity testing improves with an increase in the time allowed for observation.

Vernier acuity, also known as hyperacuity, is associated with several important characteristics:

- Vernier acuity is considered a visual cortical function rather than a retinal function.
- The accuracy of alignment in Vernier acuity is relatively resistant to optical blur. Consequently, it has been observed that Vernier acuity remains unaffected by image degradation, such as defocus or blurring, as well as motion and changes in luminance.
- Misalignments detected in Vernier acuity testing are often smaller than the diameter and spacing of retinal receptors.
- Vernier acuity is susceptible to practice effects and changes in attention. Following training, observers' thresholds have been demonstrated to improve significantly, up to six-fold.
- In peripheral vision, Vernier acuity decreases more rapidly than grating acuity.

The clinical significance of Vernier acuity lies in its ability to assess macular function in individuals with compromised optics. For instance, patients with cataracts may exhibit good Vernier acuity even in the presence of reduced normal visual acuity. This highlights the integrity of the macula, particularly when obtaining a clear view of it is challenging.

In the realm of sports, Vernier acuity holds particular relevance, especially in target sports. It contributes to understanding the visual system's mechanisms in achieving a high degree of accuracy. The Vernier acuity test simulates the target as seen through a rifle foresight, illustrating how fine judgment can be impacted by poor vision. While not a diagnostic measure of visual performance, it opens opportunities for discussion when athletes discover a significant reduction in their Vernier acuity.

ACCOMMODATION-VERGENCE FUNCTION

In the context of sports, the ability to focus clearly and rapidly on objects of regard, whether stationary object like the foresight or rear sight of the rifle while shooting or moving object like a football is crucial for athletes. Any deficit in the eyes' ability to accommodate can lead to increased effort in focusing and tracking objects, potentially slowing down response times and affecting performance, especially during long competitions where fatigue can impact the focusing muscles of the eyes.

Vergence, also known as eye teaming ability or binocularity, refers to the coordinated movement of both eyes in opposite directions to achieve or maintain single binocular vision. In sports, speed, accuracy, and sustained fusional ability are essential. For instance, quick fusional flexibility is necessary in sports like ice hockey, where players need to track fast-moving pucks. Conversely, long sustained fusional flexibility is critical in golf, where players repeatedly shift focus between the ball and the hole on the putting green. Convergence insufficiency has been seen as a cause of late braking in Formula 1 racing, resulting in excessive speed going into corners. In chess because of the intense concentration, the players have the tendency to be esophoric. In sports like snooker, long-sustained vergence facility is vital as players constantly need to converge onto the cue stick, cue ball, and target hole.

Accommodation and vergence functions are closely linked. Changes in focus automatically trigger changes in vergence and accommodation, known as the accommodation-vergence reflex. Accommodation vergence facility facilitates the eye's ability to focus clearly and accurately at different distances, relying on good oculomotor control and cognitive ability.

Accommodation and vergence functions have a great bearing on the fundamental visual skills of aiming and anticipation. In tennis, the player who is serving needs to focus on the immediate target and then on the opponent's position at the opposite end to place his shot. The receiver, on the other hand, has to focus on the server's racket, his body movement, and then the fast-approaching ball. The player has to have the ability to shift focus rapidly throughout the contest, even when general body stamina is running down due to heavy work. Poor focusing ability will severely affect anticipation. Downhill Skiing is a fast sport, and it requires fast eyes. Shifting of focus from far to near, from infinity to intermediate distance, must be efficient. As the skier becomes aware of the terrain in front and at the gates, other skiers, and trees, slow shifting of focus will delay processing for quick decision-making. The demand increases with higher speeds and more difficult terrain. In table tennis, the accommodative mechanism has to work very fast as the athlete quickly shifts his focus from near to far or intermediate targets throughout the contest. In rifle shooting, good vision is important in lining up the gun's sight with the target. There are four things in the equation: the aiming eye, the rear sight, the front sight, and the target. The participant peeps through the sights and sees three circles. He has to align these circles concentrically with the target in the middle. Unlike pistols, it is important to have a clearer picture of the sights than the target in rifle shooting. Once the shot is released, the shooter must maintain the sight picture for a few seconds. A follow-through is needed to be able to see what possible errors occurred during the release of the shot.

Accommodation is the ability to change focus from near to far and vice versa. Vergence is the ability to rapidly and accurately fuse the two images from two eyes into one image when focus is changed from near to far (divergence) and from far to near (convergence). The two eyes work as a team to maintain this in all directions of gaze and also when focus changes from point to point. Any deficit in this ability, slowness or slackness, can lead to double vision, impede anticipation and reaction time, and thereby affect the performance of the athlete.

Accommodation facilities facilitate the speed of the eye to focus clearly and accurately at different distances, which depends on good oculomotor control and cognitive ability. In modern sports, downhill skiers travelling at a speed of up to 80 mph and ice hockey players trying to hit a small, dangerous puck develop eye speed to almost superhuman levels. It, therefore, appears that fast eyes and fast sports go together.

Physiologically, eye muscles are the same as leg muscles, and the physiochemical responses underlying their activity are similar. The extraocular muscles are also under the same hormonal influence as the other skeletal muscles, but they are isolated from the external rigors of training and normal physical development. The speed of muscles decreases with age, which reduces their accommodative ability. In fact, skeletal muscles are very adaptable. Their efficiency can be improved and maintained by various exercises.

■ OCULOMOTOR FUNCTION

Oculomotor skills are the neuromuscular control skills developed to point the visual system on the target and move it to either follow a moving target or jump from one object to another. Clear vision occurs when a precisely focused image of the object of regard is centered on the fovea and the accurate eye movements or oculomotor skill maintain the relationship. Several components of oculomotor system likes Fixation, Saccades, Pursuit and Vestibular and Optokinetic movements work together to ensure that the vision is clear and stable. Saccades eye movements are abrupt shifts in fixation. The subject may present the history of trouble hitting a ball, or doing poorly in an event, or poor eye-hand coordination. Pursuit eye movement refers to the movement of eye fixating a moving object. Drugs, fatigue, emotional stress and even the test anxiety may adversely affect pursuit. Pursuit eye movement is very important in sports. For example, it would be much more difficult to track a tennis ball accurately if head movements are necessary, because the gross neck muscles are not as efficient as the finely tuned extra ocular muscles. The reflexive vestibular ocular system stabilizes the eyes on a target during head movements. It generates slow eye movement in response to head movements. This is an orientational reflex not requiring visual stimuli. Optokinetic reflexes are essentially slow eye movements in response to image movement.

Fixation is an important consideration during eye movement because the eye has to be static at the end of each saccade as it holds the image of object on the fovea. Fixation needs the combined involvement of all types of eye movements. This is a well-integrated sensory- motor process where the muscles are in dynamic equilibrium. It is interesting to note that even steady fixation is not truly motionless vision, because the eye is subject to microscopic involuntary movements. This allows the retinal image to be refreshed. Any deficits can affect fixation.

In sports the ability to maintain fixation of rapidly moving object is a critical aspect for allowing visual processing of crucial information. It also enables changing fixation from one point to another rapidly and accurately in dynamic sports and is critical to maintain steady fixation in non-dynamic sports like target shooting. The accuracy of ocular alignment of the two eyes on a given target depends upon the amount of innervations exerted by each of the six extra ocular muscles in each eye that provides precise depth judgment necessary for successful sporting performance. It is likely that muscle speed decreases with age which may contribute to slower reaction time. The speed and the precision of extra ocular muscles are very important for sporting performance at the elite level. However, the need for it can vary from one sport to another.

Geraint Griffiths has categorically mentioned in his article *'Eye speed, motility and athletic potential'* that fast eyes are associated with fast sports. In modern sports like downhill skiers traveling at a speed of 80 mph and ice-hockey player trying to hit a small dangerous puck, develops the eye speed to almost superhuman levels. Physiologically eye muscles are the same as leg muscles and physiochemical response underlying their activity are similar. The problems with making comparative measurements in thigh muscles is that performance is affected by training, high repetitions which could increase the accuracy of measurement and can cause rapid fatiguing even in trained athletes. The extraocular muscles are under the same hormonal influence as the other skeletal muscles, but they are isolated from the external rigors of training and normal physical development. Therefore, he proposed that extra-ocular muscles would be better comparative measure than any other skeletal muscle. The possibility exists that, supported by the eyes' ability to fixate on measuring points, they could be used to measure speed and so predict athlete potential.

DEPTH PERCEPTION

Depth perception is a crucial skill for anticipating the distance and speed of a target, particularly in sports like tennis and squash. These sports heavily rely on depth perception and binocular visual acuity. These visual components enable athletes to anticipate the direction and velocity of the ball. With this information and proprioceptive feedback from the arm and wrist, players can angle the racket head for an effective return shot. Anticipation, driven by depth perception, precedes aiming in the sequence of actions. Any delay in this process can result in poor timing and is often associated with reduced stereopsis. In cricket it has been seen that when a player in the outfield runs to catch a ball, correct timing depends upon the correct judgement of distance and speed of approach of the ball.

Depth perception affects the anticipation skills of athletes in sports. It involves making spatial judgment regarding the distance and the speed of the ball, teammates, opponents, boundary lines and other objects. Sports like tennis, squash which are predominantly anticipatory are highly dependent on depth perception. The critical visual components in tennis are depth perception and binocular vision. With these two components the player judges the direction and speed of the approaching ball. Using this information and proprioceptive feedback from the arm and wrist, the racket head can be angled for the return shot. So aiming follows anticipation which is the result of depth perception. If there is any delay anywhere in between, shot will not be executed in time. So poor timing is also associated with poor depth perception ability.

In table tennis, the player should anticipate the ball trajectory, direction of opponent's stroke and spatial judgment of the ball in a short time. Also peripheral judgment of environment and opponent's pattern of play have to be anticipated. So to accomplish the task successfully the perception of depth has to be of high quality.

Anticipation by depth perception is the primary skill for the batsman who anticipates the speed and direction of ball to hit. The batsman needs to develop the spatial judgment of the ball so that he can time his shot correctly. A delay in judgement will result in delay in executing the shot.

Depth perception is very important to know the spatial location of the ball and judge its relative position and direction of it fall in the air while catching. When a player runs to catch a high ball in the outfield, correct timing depends a lot upon correct judgement of distance and speed of the approach of the ball.

Depth perception is very critical for all positions in football. The spatial position of ball, efficient and accurate perception of speed and direction of ball trajectory determines the timing for eye/hand/body and foot response. The ability to pass the ball out of the reach of a defender and into the goalpost is an example of depth perception skill in football. Often the player needs to anticipate the ball in the air and makes his position accordingly to receive it.

Anticipation by depth perception is also important in highly visually demanding sports like snooker and golf. In snooker, the player focuses at the end of the cue stick, the cue ball and aims the ball at which he is shooting. Then he anticipates the distance from the hole where he intends to pot into. In golf anticipation by depth perception is needed to judge the distance between the ball and the fairway and then between the ball and the hole while putting.

Depth perception is also important in aiming predominant sports like archery as it helps the archer judge the distance of the target and then decides the extent to which the string is to be drawn. The ability allows archers to adjust their aim and determine the appropriate tension on the bowstring. Without accurate depth perception, archers may consistently misjudge distances, leading to inaccurate shots. By honing their depth perception skills, archers can improve their accuracy and performance on the field.

The ability of an athlete to block, hit or avoid a rapidly moving ball is dependent on the ability to anticipate the expected trajectory of the ball. Having quick reflex may not necessarily play a significant role. The sensory input of how quickly the image of the ball moves from eyes to brain is difficult to improve, being predominantly genetic. But how quickly the brain processes the information to the body can be dramatically improved with training. When the motor response time is quickened the athlete has more time to make a decision as to what to do with the ball.

There are various types of tests available for checking stereopsis or depth judgment. In the context of sport vision, the closer we simulate the game type condition, the more effective the results would be. Bassin Anticipation Timer is a good test developed to check the anticipation and the depth judgement ability of the athletes. The equipment allows the ability of the athlete to judge the speed of approach of an object to be measured. The ability to judge the distance and speed of a moving object as it approaches requires active accommodation, good vergence facility, visual acuity, binocular coordination which ultimately affects anticipation timing.

BINOCULAR VISION

Binocular vision encompasses the coordinated movement of the eyes and the integration of their respective views, allowing us to perceive depth and engage in detailed visual processing. Sporting performance relies heavily on well-established binocular vision, which not only affects immediate performance but also influences anticipation based on depth judgment. When binocular vision is compromised, athletes may experience a loss of confidence and inhibited muscle development due to inefficient sport participation.

In tennis, for instance, experiments blurring the vision in the non-dominant eye revealed significant impacts on players' ability to accurately hit fast-approaching spinning balls. Dominant eyes can overwhelm non-dominant ones, leading to effectively monocular vision and inhibiting depth perception and anticipation.

Similarly, in aiming sports like shooting and archery, dominant—eye athletes can often shoot without closing their non-dominant eye, as the brain naturally suppresses input from the non-dominant eye. Keeping both eyes open maximizes acuity, contrast sensitivity, depth perception, and peripheral awareness while preventing eye muscle fatigue.

Research conducted by the Sportvision group highlighted a case where an archer's slightly short-sighted dominant eye caused blurred vision during aiming, leading the brain to rely on the non-dominant eye. Unfortunately, the non-dominant eye was misaligned with the peep sight, resulting in shots consistently veering left of the target. This issue was rectified by using a -0.75 D soft contact lens in the dominant eye, restoring clear vision and improving shooting accuracy.

CENTRAL-PERIPHERAL AWARENESS

Central awareness refers to the focused attention on the central part of the visual field, where the primary action or target is located. In sports like archery or shooting, central awareness directs the athlete's attention to the bull's eye or target. It helps in maintaining focus and precision during aiming, ensuring that the athlete's aim remains centered and accurate.

Peripheral awareness involves being cognizant of the environment surrounding one's central focus. It extends beyond the direct line of vision, allowing athletes to remain alert to potential threats or opportunities from the sides. In sports like soccer or basketball, peripheral awareness enables players to anticipate the movements of opponents or teammates, facilitating quick reactions and informed decision-making. Peripheral awareness encompasses the ability to perceive actions or objects occurring outside the central line of vision. It involves maintaining awareness of objects situated to the sides while keeping focus on the central point. This skill is essential as it provides a comprehensive understanding of the surroundings, enabling timely reactions to approaching objects or individuals from the periphery. Neglecting peripheral awareness may lead to missed objects or distractions from peripheral movements, compromising safety and performance. During visual tracking, the transition from perceiving the entire field of view to focusing on a specific object is termed fixation, typically occurring within a 3-degree angle of the central visual field. Objects outside this focal point remain visible but lack detail, residing in the peripheral field. Awareness of peripheral objects, albeit out of focus, is crucial for effective navigation and overall situational awareness.

Central peripheral awareness is very important, and it affects both aiming and anticipation. In tennis, peripheral awareness aids players in monitoring both their opponent's movements and the ball's trajectory. Golf is a side-arm sport where aiming is achieved using peripheral vision to hit the ball from teeing to fairway and also while making the putt. In pole vaulting, peripheral vision helps athletes gauge the pole's position and timing throughout the event, from the approach to the final attack. The pole vaulter focuses on the box through the run up and picks up mid-mark and pole tip position using peripheral vision. Strong peripheral vision is also important to allow mid-course correction in pole tip position for efficient plant and take off timing. Yachting relies on peripheral cues such as riverbanks or lane markers for aiming, with distant marker buoys providing general course orientation. Table tennis players use peripheral awareness to anticipate opponents' movements, while badminton players must centralize their focus on the opponent's court position and on his racket and torso while simultaneously being peripheral aware of court boundaries and the net. Javelin throwers rely on peripheral vision to monitor the javelin's position and their surroundings. Archers consider peripheral factors like wind conditions when aiming, while hockey players benefit from peripheral awareness to navigate between opponents and teammates, including the goalkeeper's position. In judo, peripheral awareness enhances anticipation and reaction times during attacks and defenses. In clay pigeon shooting, central vision focuses on aiming, while peripheral awareness helps track the moving target. Maintaining visual awareness of the gun barrel's position is crucial for accurate aiming, facilitated by peripheral vision.

In some sports like boxing and motor racing, central-peripheral awareness can be life-saving. Good peripheral vision reduces injury, improves anticipation, and increases reaction speed in athletes.

Peripheral vision is affected by the speed. It is substantially reduced while running. The pathological visual field defect is caused by glaucoma, strokes, and head trauma or brain tumors. Some studies have also shown that the stress on vision also directly affects the peripheral field of vision. They discovered that as the degree of stress increases, the individual's field of vision also contracts when required to respond to a visually demanding task. Since much of what happens in sports does not happen directly in front of you, it's an important visual ability to see action on the side without having to turn your head. Nearly all sports demand good peripheral visual awareness. All ball sports require the player to localize a ball moving in their periphery quickly in order to make appropriate movement responses. The primary dictum in all sports is "keep the head as still as possible and also move the eyes as minimally as possible." It saves energy and is likely to improve performance. The split second that it takes you to change focus from an object far away to one near you may delay your reaction time and cause you to drop a pass or miss an easy volley.

Some studies indicate that athletes may be unaware of deficiencies in their peripheral vision, impacting their performance in specific areas of the game. For instance, a badminton player may struggle with high backhand shots due to delayed perception of the shuttlecock. While both the coach and player may recognize this weakness, the use of a peripheral awareness trainer can objectively identify and address the issue. Peripheral awareness proves particularly crucial in badminton, especially for high tossed returns and awareness of the partner's position and racket in doubles matches. Training in peripheral awareness can help athletes improve their overall performance and address specific challenges in their game.

In driving, peripheral vision plays a critical role in vehicle control and hazard detection. When drivers check the rear-view mirror, they rely on peripheral vision to monitor lane boundaries. Impairment of peripheral vision due to vision conditions can lead to failure in reacting to hazards from the far left or right, disregarding stoplights above intersections, or driving too closely to parked cars. Peripheral vision in driving serves to detect crucial information like road signs, hazards, and changes in traffic flow, contributing to safe driving practices. When drivers perceive something significant, they utilize head and eye movements to shift the visual focus to the central portion of their visual field, directing attention to the object or event of interest.

In cricket, maintaining good peripheral awareness is crucial, especially during moments when multiple players may converge to catch a ball, risking collisions due to intense focus on the ball. Similarly, in volleyball, players must simultaneously track the ball while being aware of teammates' and opponents' positions to optimize game play. In football, peripheral awareness often surpasses visual acuity in importance. Players rely on peripheral vision to assess the positional relationships among teammates and opponents, identify open receivers, navigate the field's boundaries, and gauge the goalkeeper's position. Defensive backs in football exemplify the use of peripheral awareness, as they primarily focus on the attacker using central vision while simultaneously monitoring the overall pattern of attack through peripheral vision.

Central vision is no doubt important, but so is the way in which peripheral awareness interacts with the central vision. In many sports, not only is peripheral awareness key to competitive ability, but it can be directly affected by deficiencies in central vision. Any residual uncorrected refractive error will tend to diminish visual performance and make the athlete less peripherally aware. The visual system tends to concentrate on the most important aspect and usually priority is given to foveal fixation. The evolutionary reason for this is that the immediate danger is in front, and secondary danger from objects approaching from sides.

To improve peripheral vision, athletes can utilize high base curve lenses and contact lenses. These measures enhance overall visual performance and contribute to better awareness of the surrounding environment during sports activities. Contact lenses offer significant advantages for athletes, particularly in enhancing peripheral awareness. Unlike spectacle lenses, contact lenses eliminate disruptive prismatic effects caused by eye movements behind fixed prescription lenses. Additionally, contact lenses eliminate potential issues associated with loosely fitting or distorted spectacle frames. Protective plano lenses in a wrap construction can safeguard against trauma without compromising peripheral awareness.

EYE-HAND-BODY COORDINATION

Eye-hand-body coordination **(Fig. 4.3)** is fundamental to sports performance, where the eyes lead and the body follows in response to visual cues. This coordination begins developing early in life and can be further honed through various exercises. It involves the synchronization of hand, feet, body, and other muscles based on information gathered through the eyes.

In fast-moving sports, such as basketball or tennis, precise eye-hand coordination and quick body movements in response to visual stimuli are critical for success. Athletes must be acutely aware of their entire body and understand the relationship between its various parts to execute movements effectively.

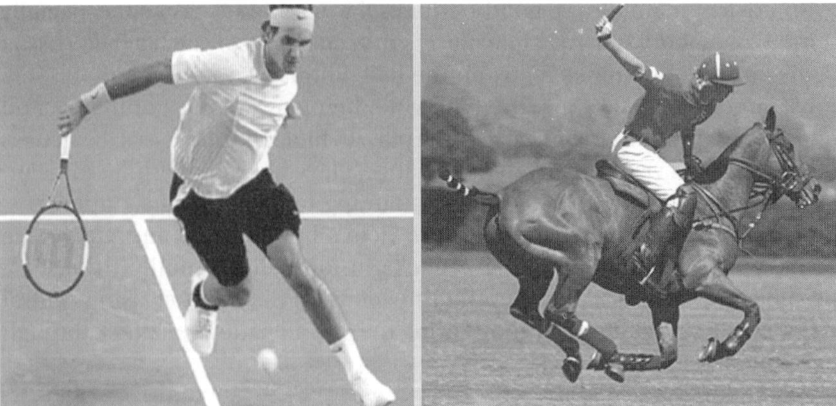

Fig. 4.3: Eye-hand-body coordination.

Central to body awareness is recognizing the body's center, while understanding the opponent's position in relation to one's own is crucial for effective response. Peripheral awareness plays a key role here, as it helps athletes gauge their surroundings and make informed decisions based on the positions of opponents and teammates. Overall, good eye-hand-body coordination is indispensable for athletes across different sports, as it influences timing, control, and responsiveness to dynamic game situations. **Figure 4.3** vividly illustrates how various bodily organs respond to stimuli encountered in sports, elucidating the significance of eye-hand-body coordination.

GLARE RECOVERY

Glare is a visual perception created when external light scatters within the eye. Glare casts a hazy veil over the retinal surface and thus significantly impairs visual acuity, contrast sensitivity, and depth perception, crucial elements for optimal sports performance **(Fig. 4.4)**.

It may occur in the presence of an extremely bright direct light source like the sun or lighting luminaries, and it can also occur because of light that bounces off a shiny surface such as a lake, wet road, snow, or glasses. Ocular media opacities also cause light scattering within the eye, resulting in glare. Studies have shown an individual's age and eye color also contributes to glare. Hypopigmentation in the iris and retina, aberrations from a large pupil, or fluorescence of blue and UV light in the ocular media. In sports, glare can be caused by stadium light, camera flashes from spectators, the surrounding environment, excessive sunlight, luminaire arrangements, etc.

The effect of glare often results in:
- Eye squinting
- Headaches
- Visual fatigue

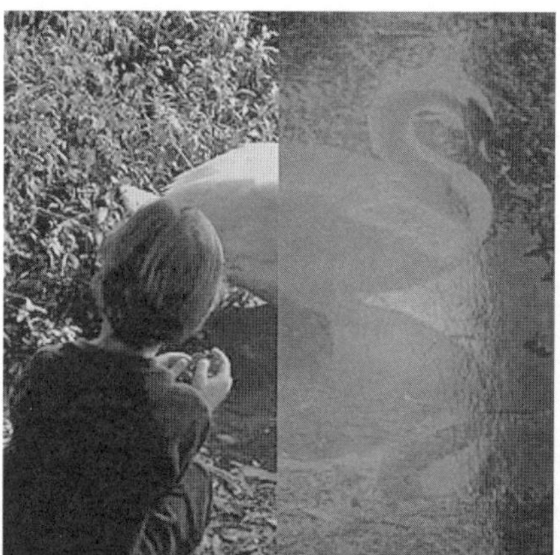
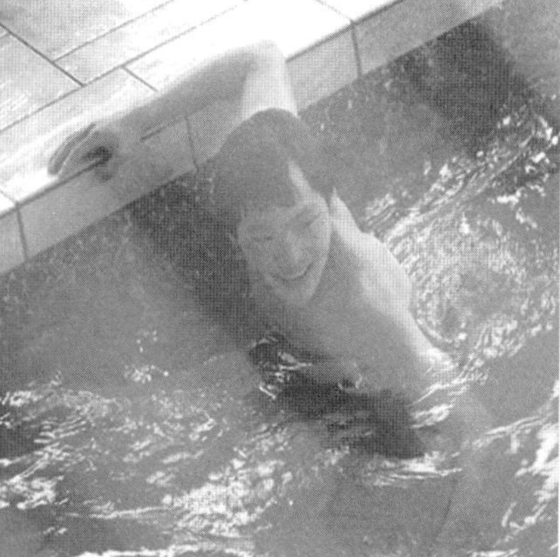

Fig. 4.4: Effect of glare.

- Eye strain
- Reduced vision
- Reduced contrast
- Poor color perception
- It affects an athlete's ability to focus and maintain concentration during training sessions and competitions.

Glare problems are often seen as a serious threat to the performance of athletes. The effect of glare seems to be difficult to eliminate. However, it can be minimized by good lighting arrangements, protective eyewear, and individualized glare management strategies.

In sports where high-speed movements and precise coordination are essential, impaired vision due to glare can pose serious safety risks to athletes and others on the field. Ensuring quick glare recovery helps athletes react swiftly to sudden changes in the environment and avoid potential accidents. Glare recovery is the time taken to recover from the effects of disability glare. Poor glare recovery may lead to compromised depth perception and spatial awareness, increasing the likelihood of collisions, falls, or misjudgments during sports activities. By optimizing glare recovery, athletes can better assess their surroundings and minimize the risk of injury, enabling them to stay focused, alert, and mentally resilient throughout the duration of the game or training session.

Glare recovery time assessment provides valuable insights into athletes' visual function, including their ability to recover from glare-induced visual impairment. By measuring how quickly athletes regain optimal visual clarity after exposure to glare, coaches, trainers, and eye care professionals can assess the efficiency of their visual system.

Optimizing glare recovery time contributes to improved performance and safety outcomes in sports. Athletes with shorter glare recovery times are better equipped to maintain clear vision, react quickly to changing game dynamics, and minimize the risk of visual distractions or impairments that could compromise their performance or safety on the field or court.

Sportvision Practice: Scope

5 CHAPTER

A clear distinction exists between general optometry practice and sports vision practice. In general optometry, individuals typically visit optometrists due to visual, ocular, or reflective symptoms, or as part of routine eye care. Optometrists conduct examinations using standard equipment in an environment conducive to visual acuity testing, often prescribing corrections to achieve 20/20 or 6/6 vision on the Snellen chart. The interaction mainly revolves around symptom management, and unless symptoms persist, the interaction is usually brief.

In contrast to general optometry practice, sports vision practice takes a markedly different approach. Athletes often exhibit above-average vision and may not perceive the necessity for visual intervention. The objective of sports vision optometry is to assess athletes' visual efficiency and correlate any deficiencies detected with their sporting performance and advocate for vision training where necessary. Vision, in the context of sports vision is much more than the ability to read the 20/20 line in the test chart. It includes many other faculties like eye movements, depth perception, peripheral awareness, focusing ability, fixation, and visual reaction time and so on. Coordination, concentration, balance and accuracy are a few other visually-related abilities that are critical during a sporting event. Athletes believe that although they need eyesight examination, but their eyesight is good and hence they don't accept easily if some visual deficiency is detected. The sportvision practitioner must demonstrate the deficiency and explain its relation to his sporting performance to motivate the athlete to follow his advice. Athlete engagement is pivotal in this process, fostering understanding and collaboration towards improving visual performance.

The principle guiding sports vision practice underscores the pivotal role of the eyes in supplying information to the brain, which subsequently orchestrates motor responses. The accuracy and speed of this information processing profoundly impact athletic performance.

The scope of sports vision practice adapts to the varying needs of athletes at different levels:

- Aspiring athletes embark on vision training early in their athletic journey, integrating visual skill development into their training regimens to augment proficiency and readiness for competitive endeavors.
- Elite athletes, on the other hand, pursue advanced techniques and strategies within sports vision practice. They aim to refine their visual abilities to gain a competitive advantage and ascend to exceptional levels of performance, continuously striving for excellence in their athletic pursuits.

In summary, sports vision practice tailor interventions to meet athletes' specific needs, emphasizing collaboration between practitioners, coaches, managers, and athletes themselves to optimize visual performance and enhance overall athletic prowess.

WORKING WITH EARLY STARTERS

In the real world, individuals often exhibit distinct strengths and weaknesses across various activities, prompting inquiry into the factors behind these differences. It is widely believed that both nature and nurture play significant roles in shaping individual aptitudes, with innate abilities predisposing individuals to certain sports while environmental factors, motivation, and opportunities contribute to their engagement in specific activities. The visual characteristics of an athlete may strongly influence their choice of sport, with certain visual behaviors aligning with particular sports requirements.

For instance, in cricket, left eye dominance in a right-handed player may favor fast bowling but pose challenges in batting. Ideally, right-handed archers should have right eye dominance to facilitate accurate aiming. Similarly, right eye dominance may predispose individuals to excel in rifle shooting. Recognizing such predispositions can inform the early assessment of visual skills through sports vision optometry, enabling tailored recommendations and interventions from the outset of an athlete's career.

Moreover, individuals born with visual disadvantages may harness their challenges as potent motivators, driving them to excel in their chosen sport. Soccer, for instance, demands acute peripheral awareness, suggesting that individuals with reduced central vision may thrive in the sport by adapting to their visual deficiencies and enhancing peripheral awareness.

Furthermore, the speed and precision of extraocular muscles play a crucial role in modern sports performance. These muscles, akin to skeletal muscles, exhibit speed and accuracy in eye movements, which can serve as indicators of an athlete's potential. Research has shown that fast eyes and fast sports go together. It could be interesting to know at the early stage based on which a configuration could be derived.

Initiating sports vision training at the onset of an athlete's career offers insights into their natural abilities and allows for tailored recommendations based on comprehensive eye examinations. For example, a right-handed batsman with left-eye dominance experiencing inconsistent performance may benefit from trying left-handed batting, leveraging their dominant eye for improved accuracy and performance. It is easier to train the body to bat left-handed than to change eye dominance. Initially the feeling may be lack of power, but confidence would grow quickly as the ball began to hit the middle of the bat.

In conclusion, refining and improvising early sports vision training can unlock athletes' potential, optimize their performance, and pave the way for success in their chosen sports endeavors.

■ WORKING AT ELITE LEVEL

At the elite level of sports, athletes' abilities alone are no longer the primary factors determining success. While sporting prowess remains relatively consistent among athletes, factors such as fitness, speed, strategy, sleep quality, mental and emotional conditions have emerged as critical differentiators. The landscape of competition has evolved, becoming increasingly intense and demanding. In such a competitive environment, athletes are constantly seeking elusive advantages over their rivals, and vision stands out as one such factor.

Vision plays a pivotal role in sporting performance, serving as the primary source of information acquisition. Over 80% of information is obtained through vision, and quicker visual processing allows athletes more time to react effectively. Delays in receiving visual information can lead to slower response times and potentially inadequate performance outcomes.

Despite the critical importance of vision at the highest levels of competition, scientifically correlating visual performance with sporting achievements proves challenging due to numerous variables such as coaching, environmental conditions, opponents, and overall health. Nevertheless, the potential for improvement in visual skills remains substantial.

At this level of practice, sports vision optometrists may transition into roles as sport vision consultants for individual athletes or professional teams, establishing comprehensive sport vision clinics for vision training. The hypothesis suggests that the distinction between a good player and a great player is often minimal; highlighting the critical role that sports vision professionals can play as specialized trainers. Research indicates that even minor visual deficiencies in one eye can significantly impact an athlete's performance at the elite level.

Problems with visual processing, if left unaddressed, can profoundly affect an athlete's performance. Instances such as consistently hitting the front of the rim in basketball or overshooting the golf hole may stem from underlying vision issues rather than athletic ability alone. Compensating for visual weaknesses can lead to the development of vulnerabilities in an athlete's game, which opponents may exploit during competition. Consultant sports vision specialists are adept at identifying and addressing such weaknesses, working collaboratively with athletes to treat visual deficiencies and optimize performance outcomes.

Sports vision has its foundations in behavioral optometry, which explores the connection between visual performance and occupation. Like many other professions, sports can be viewed as an occupation, albeit one with an exceptionally high level of visual demand, especially in competitive settings. Occupations involve how individuals interact with their environment and navigate through the world. One of the primary limitations of general optometry practice has been the oversight regarding the relevance of vision to occupation-specific tasks. The objective of sports vision practice goes beyond identifying visual defects; it aims to assess the efficiency of the visual system and establish a direct link between visual deficiencies and an athlete's performance in their sport. This paradigm shift elevates the importance of refraction as a diagnostic tool and assessment method.

The practice of sports vision necessitates a collaborative effort among coaches, managers, players, and practitioners. Managers play a crucial role in ensuring that their teams undergo regular vision screenings. Many individuals, including athletes, may be unaware of their underperforming vision, leading to missed opportunities for improvement.

Contrary to common belief, vision significantly influences sporting performance at all levels, including elite competitions where the implications can be profound, both in terms of performance and commercial outcomes. While athletes diligently train their aerobic capacity, strength, and flexibility, vision often gets overlooked. However, the eyes are integral to the body's physiological system, leading in all actions and reactions. Whether tracking a flying ball, returning a serve, throwing a pass, or aiming for a target, the eyes take the lead, guiding the rest of the body. Neglecting eye health and visual training can hinder overall performance. Therefore, incorporating vision care and training into athletes' routines is essential for optimizing their potential and enhancing their competitive edge on the field.

In sports vision practice, athletes typically present with either peak visual acuity or near-peak visual acuity. They are more concerned with understanding how their visual system impacts their sporting abilities and whether any deficiencies can be corrected through vision training. Therefore, the key lies in demonstrating the status of their visual system so that athletes can comprehend the implications and collaborate with practitioners to design appropriate vision correction and training programs. This process often involves multiple sessions, conducted either in a sports vision clinic, on the field, or with coaches. It is important for practitioners to avoid treating athletes as patients since they are otherwise healthy individuals with good vision. Athletes are partners in the process, and their feedback, whether positive or negative, is essential for refining the approach.

Historically, individuals who prioritize wearing full correction and undergo regular eye check-ups tend to have better visual performance potential. This underscores the importance of vision in competitive sports preparation, surpassing other physiological characteristics like muscle size and physical stature. Athletes need to recognize that a visual assessment cannot worsen their performance but holds significant potential for improvement. Club officials should understand that visual assessment aims to enhance the squad's strength and depth by identifying areas for improvement rather than eliminating players who need assistance. There's a misconception that sports vision is distinct from mainstream optometry, but in reality, it encompasses various aspects, from routine refraction to safety considerations and pathological assessments, contributing significantly to athletes' performance and well-being.

Researchers have demonstrated that at the elite level of sports competition, the physical preparation, strength, speed, stamina, agility, and skill levels of the top performers are often similar. The distinguishing factor between a superb player and a great player lies in the speed of their vision. Gold medalists in highly competitive events typically possess superior balance, precision, and exceptional visual abilities. Their ability to perceive and interpret visual stimuli quickly enables them to react with speed and accuracy.

Sports vision addresses these critical visual skills, which often receive less attention from coaches and team managers. Vision is an athlete's intangible asset, serving as the initial step in information processing. Clear and complete visual input is essential for optimal reaction and performance across various sports disciplines. In track and field, golf, cricket, football, car racing, tennis, shooting, and other sports, inadequate visual processing can result in timing issues, missed shots, poor passes, late braking, and other performance challenges.

At the international level of competition where elite athletes vie for gold, the margin between victory and defeat is minuscule. While athletes possess core skills and undergo rigorous physical conditioning, they often overlook the importance of vision. However, the eyes play a crucial role in every action and reaction, and neglecting visual conditioning can hinder overall performance. In today's fiercely competitive environment, even a single mistake or delayed reaction can jeopardize an athlete's career.

Vision training is essential for enhancing visual skills such as eye coordination, focusing ability, and eye-hand coordination, thereby reducing reaction time and improving performance. Great athletes in highly competitive sports likely possess exceptional visual abilities, complementing their technical skills, equipment, diet, physical training, and mental endurance. Evaluating potential visual problems and addressing deficiencies through sports vision practice can unlock hidden potential and level the playing field.

While vision training cannot single-handedly guarantee athletic success, it serves to remove visual barriers and enhance performance. Combining vision training with physical conditioning can yield unbeatable results, making vision training the final frontier for athletes seeking to elevate their performance.

INDICATIONS OF VISION PROBLEMS AFFECTING SPORTS PERFORMANCE

Vision encompasses intricate connections between the eyes, brain, and muscles, facilitating the interpretation of three-dimensional phenomena through fusion. Continuous eye movements scan the visual field until attention is captured, a process known as fixation. Fixations are crucial as the focus ability is limited to a very small area of the visual field, highlighting the significance of peripheral vision in sports. Peripheral information aids in quick motion detection, enabling redirection of visual focus to other events. Athletes' eye movements have been analyzed to understand visual search strategies, if fixations reflect perceptual decision-making strategies.

Good eyesight is vital for motor skills like catching a ball or contacting with a bat, while also influencing tactical elements such as player movement and shot selection. Visual information underpins spatial orientation, anticipation, timing, reactions, and balance, guiding effective anticipation and decision-making during games. While factors like skill, fitness, fatigue, environment, knowledge, and training impact athletes' decision-making, vision takes precedence.

Recent research in sport vision underscores that clear and accurate vision significantly impacts performance across various sports. Athletes rely on their eyes to lead their bodies, and the stamina, flexibility, and fine-tuning of the visual system provide split-second timing needed for excellence. Compensation for deficient visual skills may result in weak spots in sporting ability, exploited by opponents in competitive scenarios.

In today's fiercely competitive sporting world, where a single mistake can derail a career, good vision parallels the importance of physical conditioning and mental focus. Visual conditioning is gaining recognition, given its crucial role in enhancing athletic performance. Studies indicate that athletes often exhibit superior visual abilities compared to the general population, showcasing enhanced focus flexibility, depth perception, eye-hand coordination, and anticipation. The correlation between fast eyes and fast sports further emphasizes the pivotal role of vision in athletic excellence.

Indeed, at the elite level, good vision can be the distinguishing factor between a good athlete and an exceptional one. Athletes may exhibit certain performance indicators signaling potential areas for improvement in their sporting performance by addressing their visual system:

- Despite possessing top-quality sporting equipment and demonstrating exceptional skills, the athlete fails to perform up to their potential.
- The athlete consistently makes the same errors or faults despite taking corrective measures.
- Additional coaching or practice fails to yield desired results for the athlete.
- The athlete struggles to track the ball or other players during play.
- There are instances of overestimating or underestimating distances, affecting performance in activities like short putts in golf or late braking in car racing.
- Concentration issues lead to inconsistent performance, such as missing gold in shooting competitions.
- The athlete's reactions appear slower than optimal.
- Frequent missed catches, poor passes, or inadequate returns in tennis indicate visual processing challenges.
- Batsmen frequently miss shots during cricket matches.

Identifying and addressing these performance indicators related to visual skills can potentially elevate an athlete's performance from good to exceptional.

Many elite-level athletes overlook the potential impact of vision on their performance, often believing their eyesight to be flawless and unrelated to their sporting abilities. This misconception poses a significant barrier to encouraging athletes to undergo vision examinations. Bridging the gap between athletes and coaches is essential in addressing this issue. One effective approach is engaging athletes in discussions and demonstrating how various aspects of their visual system can influence their performance in their respective sports.

A sportvision optometrist must approach sports from the perspective of an optometrist, possessing a deep understanding of various sports and their dynamics. Actively participating in sporting events, studying training tapes, interacting with coaches, and staying informed through sports literature are crucial for performance analysis. Establishing rapport with athletes is paramount, enabling the optometrist to work closely with them as personal trainers rather than treating them as patients. Athletes visiting sportvision optometrists seek not immediate remedial treatment but rather guidance for enhancing their performance. Therefore, terms like "patient" and "deficiency" may not resonate with them. Instead, presenting vision assessment results as "strengths" and "opportunities" can be more effective, emphasizing areas for improvement rather than shortcomings.

It is important to recognize that the muscles of the eyes, like other muscles in the body, can be conditioned and improved with the help of sportvision specialists. Just as physical trainers work on strengthening muscles to enhance physical performance, sportvision specialists focus on optimizing the efficiency of the visual system to improve overall athletic performance.

PREVENTION AND PROTECTION

Optometry has traditionally focused on detecting pathology, but the preventive aspect of optometry has not always been clear or emphasized. However, optimal enjoyment of life is closely tied to good health and well-being. Good health encompasses the proper functioning of all bodily organs, and each aspect of health is interconnected. The eyes, as part of the physiological system, are susceptible to various environmental factors that can impact their health.

Studies have highlighted the detrimental effects of non-ionizing radiation on the eyes, particularly contributing to conditions like cataracts and macular degeneration. Additionally, the soft tissues around the eyes are vulnerable to sunlight, increasing the risk of conditions like basal and squamous cell carcinoma, as well as pinguecula and pterygium due to overexposure.

The philosophy of eye protection revolves primarily around avoidance. Eye injuries are a significant concern, especially in fast-paced and dynamic activities. Many studies have underscored the importance of eye protection, particularly in sports where the risk of traumatic eye injuries is high. These injuries can range from blowout fractures of the orbit to tears in the iris, retinal detachment, and penetrating eye injuries.

Unfortunately, humans often take their vision for granted. However, wearing well-designed sunglasses can provide protection against various hazards, including impacts from particles and insects, exposure to pollen and wind, and harmful UV radiation. Choosing lenses that offer complete UV protection is essential for safeguarding eye health.

In summary, it is crucial to prioritize eye protection to prevent potential visual disabilities that could impact one's quality of life. Investing in protective eyewear is a proactive measure that can help maintain optimal eye health and prevent long-term damage.

MAINTENANCE OF SIGHT

The vision enhancement side of optometry says that vision and sporting performance are directly linked. Vision has profound implications on the ability of an athlete to perform. This automatically establishes the importance of its maintenance. The good vision or the enhanced vision, if not maintained, cannot provide a long sporting life to the athlete. People who play sports for longer because they are visually able to, will also be extending the useful life of their eyesight. One thing intimately depends on the other. One of the main aspects of sports that they are often played outside during all sorts of weather conditions, including bright sunlight or conditions where there are strong reflections from the ground or from water or from the surroundings. There is lot of evidence that non-ionizing radiation contributes to an aging effect in the eye, specially cataract and macular degeneration.

Cataract

It is well accepted that shorter wavelengths of light are more damaging due to the higher energy contained in each photon. Despite this, blue eyes tend to be more susceptible to macular degeneration, while brown eyes are more prone to cataracts. The primary reason for this may be related to the effects of heat and the lower energy associated with longer wavelengths, such as red and infrared light.

Dark irises, like those in brown eyes, absorb heat more readily than pale blue irises and act as heat sinks since they sit over the lens of the eye. This suggests that environmentally induced cataracts may occur because the dark iris "cooks" the underlying lens, similar to how an egg cooks in a hot frying pan.

Additionally, the location of posterior subcapsular cataracts, which coincide with the nodal point of the lens through which all energy is focused, supports the idea that tissues exposed to continuous energy are more susceptible to degeneration. This makes them more prone to cataracts over time.

Macular Degeneration

The ocular media absorb higher wavelengths of light, making macular problems from infrared radiation unlikely. Most UV rays are also absorbed before reaching the retina, but UV radiation between 380 to 400 nm (where UV becomes blue light) can reach the retina.

Each photon of light that lands on the retina causes bleaching in the rods and cones, increasing the metabolic demand to regenerate pigments. This process produces metabolic by-products that must be cleared by the blood system. Overexposure to intense sunlight, especially from reflective surfaces, can overwhelm this clearance process, leading to the build-up of macular drusen. Drusen form a barrier between photoreceptor cells and underlying vascular tissues.

When tissues are deprived of oxygen, they release chemical messengers to stimulate new blood vessel formation. These new vessels form under the macula in a circular pattern and are prone to leaking plasma and blood, leading to macular detachment and degeneration.

This strongly supports the clinical importance of dispensing because the right use of lens materials and filters can prevent the occurrence of cataract and macular degeneration.

HAZARDS OF NON-IONIZING RADIATIONS

Non-ionizing radiation refers to a type of electromagnetic radiation that does not have enough energy to ionize atoms or molecules. These forms of electromagnetic radiation as shown in **Figure 5.1** have wavelengths that vary across the electromagnetic spectrum and do not carry enough energy to ionize atoms or molecules.

Ultraviolet Radiations

Ultraviolet (UV) radiation spans from approximately 380 nanometers into the lower regions of the electromagnetic spectrum. UV rays represent the shorter wavelength end of the spectrum and pose greater potential for damaging the eyes. The level of damage is contingent upon the intensity of the energy reaching the ocular tissues and the duration of exposure. Any part of the eye or its surrounding structures impacted by shorter wavelength radiation is vulnerable. Those areas responsible for focusing light are particularly susceptible, such as the nodal point of the lens and the fovea.

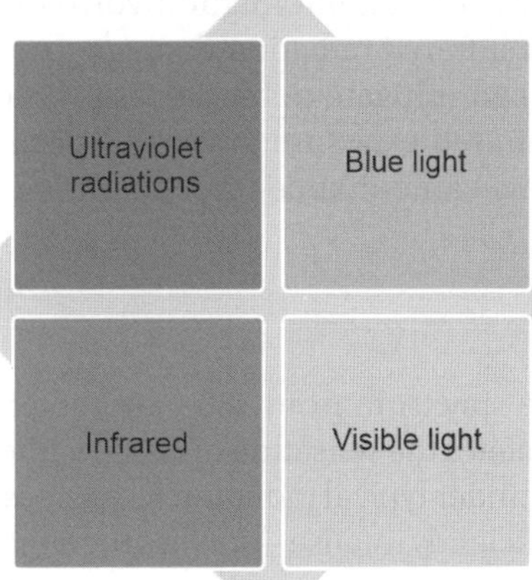

Fig. 5.1: Non-ionizing radiations.

The posterior subcapsular cataract, situated near the nodal point, is especially affected by UV exposure. However, the ocular media, including the cornea and lens, exhibit strong UV absorption, thereby reducing its impact on the retina. Only a small portion of the UV spectrum, specifically between 380 nanometers and 400 nanometers, reaches the macula, which is of particular concern for eye health.

Refinement and improvement may involve providing more context on the risks associated with UV exposure, such as the development of cataracts, macular degeneration, and other ocular conditions. Additionally, discussing preventive measures like wearing UV-protective sunglasses and avoiding prolonged exposure to UV rays can enhance the comprehensiveness of the information provided.

Infrared Radiations

The region above 780 nanometers is categorized as the infrared end of the electromagnetic spectrum. Radiant energy from the infrared region has thermal effects, the extent of which depends on the intensity and duration of exposure. Over 90% of the incident infrared radiation energy is absorbed by ocular structures such as the cornea, iris, lens, and vitreous, with only a small percentage reaching the retina. Consequently, all eye tissues can be affected by infrared radiation.

Despite its significance, infrared radiation has often been overlooked, although it has been associated with conditions like glass blower's cataract. An intriguing aspect is the relationship between cataracts and macular degeneration. If non-ionizing radiation is the cause of macular degeneration, then absorption of this radiation by the lens, resulting in sclerosis, might actually prevent macular changes.

It appears that eyes which allow light to penetrate more easily are at greater risk of macular degeneration due to exposure to non-ionizing radiations. Refining and improving the content might involve providing more context on the mechanisms of infrared radiation damage to ocular tissues and how preventive measures can mitigate potential risks. Additionally, discussing the implications of infrared exposure in various occupational settings and everyday environments can enhance understanding and awareness of its impact on eye health.

Visible Light

Visible light spans the spectrum from 380 nanometers to 780 nanometers, where the energy stimulates the sensation of vision without causing significant harm to ocular tissues under typical radiation intensities. However, it is crucial to note that light, if sufficiently intense—such as the sunlight in Mediterranean climates during summer—can accumulate enough photons to potentially affect the retina and lens over time.

To refine and enhance the content, it might be beneficial to delve deeper into the concept of cumulative light exposure and its impact on eye health.

Explaining how excessive exposure to intense light sources, even within the visible spectrum, can lead to conditions like photokeratitis, photoconjunctivitis, and long-term damage to ocular structures can provide valuable insights. Additionally, discussing preventive measures such as wearing sunglasses, using UV-protective eyewear, and minimizing direct exposure to bright light sources can help mitigate potential risks associated with intense visible light.

Blue Light

Blue light, with a wavelength ranging from approximately 380 nm to 500 nm, is one of the shortest and highest-energy wavelengths in the visible spectrum. It is emitted by various sources including the sun and digital screens. Blue light carries a significant amount of energy per photon, making it potentially harmful to the eyes.

While natural exposure to blue light during the day can enhance energy, alertness, and mood, prolonged exposure to blue light from screens, especially during evening or nighttime, can disrupt the body's circadian rhythm and lead to various health issues, including sleep disorders.

Chronic exposure to blue light may increase the risk of early age-related macular degeneration (ARMD) and other ocular pathologies. Sunlight, particularly the high-energy light between 380 to 500 nm, is considered a factor that can cause cumulative damage to the retina.

Research from Harvard has associated working night shifts and exposure to blue light at night with several health conditions, including certain types of cancer (such as breast and prostate cancer), diabetes, heart disease, obesity, and an increased risk of depression.

Immediate effect of Blue Light is seen as glare effect together with bright light of the screen. The largest single enemy today in the digi world is the glare which may be defined as "light pollution" and the effect of which increases with time spent and also with increase in age.

Other Pathologies

In addition to cataracts and macular degeneration, there are other pathologies associated with non-ionizing radiation.

Pinguecula

Pinguecula is a small area of conjunctival degeneration which frequently occurs nasally to the limbus. It is thought that one reason for its particular location is the refraction of side incident light by the cornea. This effect can be seen clearly with a pen torch shone to the side of the eye. The focusing of the light in this area causes the typical degeneration seen in pinguecula, of a slightly raised yellowy area of tissue. This is typical of a benign lesion caused by sunlight.

Pterygium

Pterygium is an extension of conjunctival tissue onto the epithelium of the cornea, due to a breakdown in the structure of the eye at the limbus. The limbus is very important as a source of stem cells which regenerate the corneal epithelium and form a barrier between the conjunctiva and the epithelium. The breakdown of this barrier is likely to have the same etiology as the pinguecula which occurs in the same area on the eye. It is simply due to overexposure to sunlight and UV.

Basal Cell Carcinoma

It is a common form of skin cancer often associated with overexposure to UV radiation. It typically occurs in the soft tissues of the adnexa, which include the structures surrounding the eye. This malignancy is characterized by the uncontrolled growth of basal cells, which are found in the outermost layer of the skin.

SCOPE FOR SPORT VISION PRACTICE

Sport vision screening serves as the initial step in addressing athletes' visual needs and enhancing their performance on the field or court. The process involves conducting quick assessments of athletes' visual abilities in specific sporting contexts, providing immediate feedback and demonstration of the importance of vision in their particular sport. Screening protocols are designed to identify potential visual deficiencies or areas for improvement that may impact athletic performance.

The significance of sport vision screening lies in its ability to create awareness among athletes about the importance of vision in sports performance. Many athletes, despite acknowledging the importance of vision, may have never undergone an eye examination, assuming their vision to be perfect. By demonstrating how vision directly impacts their sporting performance, athletes are encouraged to take proactive steps towards addressing any identified visual issues.

Following sport vision screening, athletes who demonstrate significant visual deficiencies or require further evaluation undergo comprehensive clinical assessments in a controlled clinical setting. Clinical practice in sport vision involves a thorough examination of various aspects of visual function, including binocular vision, accommodative abilities, visual processing, and ocular health.

Optometrists working in clinical settings utilize advanced diagnostic tools and therapeutic techniques to optimize visual function and support athletes' overall visual health. They prescribe personalized treatment plans, which may include vision therapy exercises, corrective lenses, or specialized treatments tailored to address specific visual challenges or enhance visual performance in sports-specific contexts.

The sequential approach of sport vision screening followed by clinical practice ensures that athletes receive comprehensive care tailored to their individual visual needs. While screening aims to identify potential visual deficiencies and create awareness among athletes, clinical practice focuses on ongoing monitoring and management of athletes' visual health and performance.

By integrating vision screening into real sporting situations, optometrists play a vital role in maximizing athlete potential and promoting long-term success in sports. Through collaboration with athletes, coaches, and sports medicine professionals, optometrists bridge the gap between athletes and practitioners, fostering collaborative relationships aimed at optimizing athletic performance through enhanced visual skills.

Designing simpler and easy-to-administer tests for sport vision screening is crucial for motivating athletes to prioritize their visual health and incorporate sport vision training into their overall athletic development. Developing screening tests tailored to the visual demands of different sports, providing immediate feedback, and utilizing engaging and interactive methods can significantly enhance athlete participation and understanding of the importance of vision in sports. This approach ensures athletes actively engage in sport vision training as an integral part of their overall sporting development.

6 CHAPTER Sports Vision Screening

Sport vision screening is a concise eye examination program designed to identify potential areas of concern that may affect an athlete's vision and thereby sporting performance. It is not intended to diagnose vision problems or eye disorders. Indeed, if issues are detected during a vision screening program, the individual is referred to a specialist for further evaluation and treatment. The specialist conducts a comprehensive eye examination in a clinical setting using advanced tests and equipment, developing an appropriate treatment plan based on the findings.

Vision serves as the intangible asset of an athlete and acts as the initial step in information processing. Any difficulty in the vision processing mechanism can result in unclear or incomplete information reaching the brain, leading to suboptimal reactions from the athlete. This can manifest differently across various sporting events. For instance,

- In track and field, it may cause timing issues;
- In golf, short putting; in cricket, missed shots;
- In football, poor passing;
- In car racing, late braking;
- In tennis, poor returns;
- In shooting, missed targets, and so forth.

Despite corrective measures taken during sport-specific training, performance inadequacies may persist if underlying vision-related issues remain unaddressed. The objective of sport vision screening encompasses two primary goals:

- To identify any potential visual deficiencies.
- To demonstrate to the athlete how these deficiencies impact their vision performance in relation to their sporting performance.

Many elite athletes are unaware that their performance shortcomings can stem from vision issues. This is because they believe that although vision is important, their own vision is perfect. This perception creates a significant barrier. Therefore, sport vision assessments should be strategically designed and executed in two phases.

The first phase can be a sport vision screening, followed by an in-depth examination in a clinical environment. The screening program should not only identify vision-related issues but also demonstrate to athletes how their visual systems are functioning. This allows optometrists to explain the impact of these issues on sporting performance, making the relevance clear to the athletes and encouraging collaboration to design suitable vision correction and visual training programs. The greatest obstacle to seeking optometric advice is the disbelief that vision is connected to sporting performance.

Sport vision screening tests can be conducted either on-site or in a clinical environment. They should include a set of diagnostic tests and tests for specific visual skills related to the athlete's particular position in their chosen sport. Geraint proposed that these be called *analytical tests.*

DIAGNOSTIC TESTS

Geraint Griffiths has proposed six diagnostic tests that can be effectively used to achieve the sportvision screening objective. These tests break down the vision into its component parts and try to diagnose which aspect of visual performance is at fault for the individual athlete and also demonstrate why these aspects of vision are important to their sporting performance **(Fig. 6.1)**.

Retinoscopy

Retinoscopy is an objective method used to assess the refractive status of the eye relative to the point of fixation. This test does not rely on the subject's response, making it highly reliable. In screening, retinoscopy efficiently measures common refractive errors such as long-sightedness, short-sightedness, astigmatism, or discrepancies between the two eyes, all of which can significantly impact sporting performance.

During screening, retinoscopy also provides valuable insights into the ocular health of athletes. By examining the eyes, signs of pathologies such as cataracts or keratoconus can be detected early on. This comprehensive evaluation helps ensure athletes maintain optimal visual health and performance on the field or court.

High and Low Contrast Acuity

LogMAR charts have emerged as an advancement over Snellen's chart for measuring visual acuity due to their ability to provide data that can be statistically analyzed. Unlike Snellen's chart, LogMAR charts maintain a uniform relationship between the lines and the number of letters in each line. Additionally, LogMAR charts are available in both high contrast (90%) and low contrast (10%) options.

The inclusion of low contrast charts is particularly beneficial as they simulate real-life scenarios where visibility may be compromised, such as in poor light, fading sunlight, mist, rain, or when dealing with a dirty kit. Performance deficiencies under low contrast conditions can be significant, even if high contrast acuity is reasonably good. This makes low contrast testing

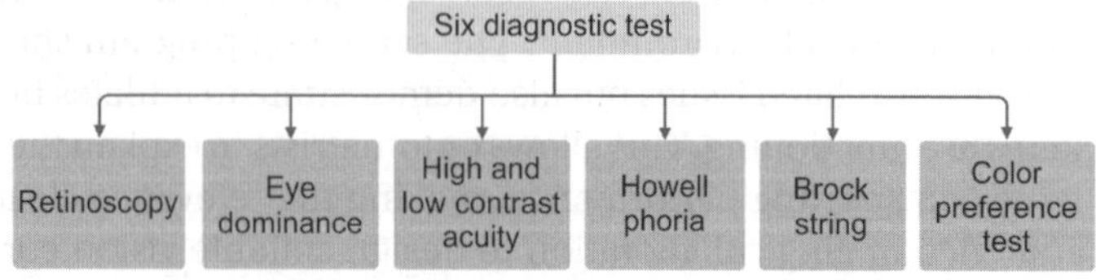

Fig. 6.1: Six diagnostic tests for sport vision screening.

especially relevant for athletes, helping to identify and address vision issues that could impact their performance in challenging environments.

During the screening process, it is crucial not only to identify visual deficiencies but also to relate these findings to the athlete's understanding of their sport and why they may pose a problem. This contextualization helps athletes grasp the importance of addressing visual acuity issues and underscores their relevance to sporting performance.

Eye Dominance

Eye dominance, although typically not assessed during routine eye examinations, holds significant importance in the context of sport vision. This test provides crucial insights into an individual's visual performance in sports and helps elucidate relationships between vision and sporting prowess that may otherwise remain obscure. Therefore, it is imperative to include eye dominance testing as a routine procedure during the screening stage of sport vision assessments.

Several compelling reasons underscore the necessity of eye dominance testing during sport vision screening. Firstly, eye dominance is sport-specific and represents an innate characteristic of individuals. Understanding an athlete's dominant eye can shed light on their predisposition towards certain sports or activities.

Furthermore, eye dominance testing aids in explaining discrepancies in visual performance that cannot be elucidated solely through standard vision assessments. By identifying the dominant eye, sport vision specialists can tailor interventions and training programs to optimize an athlete's visual skills, ultimately enhancing their performance on the field or court.

Howell Phoria

The assessment of muscle balance, crucial for understanding visual performance in athletes, traditionally involves the cover test, which can be challenging due to its reliance on subjective estimation, especially for deviations less than 3 diopters of prism.

The Howell Phoria test offers a more objective measure of muscle balance, particularly in terms of horizontal prism diopters. This test evaluates horizontal phorias at both distance and near, providing a more natural testing environment compared to the Cover test and Maddox Wing test. Athletes can actively observe their vision during the test, facilitating their understanding of the results and prompting discussions on the significance of the numbers obtained.

During the Howell Phoria test, athletes witness their performance quantified in numbers, prompting discussions on the relevance of these findings to their ability to judge distance accurately. The use of six base down prisms in front of the right eye allows for the creation of a diplopic image, enabling moment-to-moment monitoring of changes in phoria.

By the time athletes undergo a full eye examination, they arrive with questions already in mind, ready to engage in discussions about corrective measures and interventions. The Howell Phoria test serves as a valuable tool in this process, fostering athlete engagement and facilitating targeted interventions to optimize visual performance in sports.

Brock String

The Brock string serves as a powerful tool for athletes to gain insight into the intricate processes of vision. It effectively measures fixation disparity, a concept particularly relevant in sports, as it can be adjusted to various angles and positions to mimic real-life sporting scenarios. The string also detects suppression and assesses the alignment accuracy of the eyes in space.

Standard testing is done at 40 cm, 1 metre and 3 meters in all position of gaze up, down, straight depending upon the need of the sport. During screening, a single bead placed at 40 cm is often sufficient to demonstrate potential anomalies to athletes, prompting further investigation during a full eye examination. The string is anchored at one end to a fixed object while the subject holds the other end at their nose crest. The subject focuses on the bead in the middle of the string.

If both eyes are converged and focused on the bead, the subject should see double string approaching the bead, meeting at bead and a double string diverging from the point of meet forming a cross appearance. The accuracy of binocular vision is determined by the string meeting at the object of regard, i.e., making cross at the bead.

Several scenarios may arise during Brock string testing:

- If the strings appear to meet before the bead, it suggests over-convergence of the eyes and potential decompensated esophoria.
- If the strings meet beyond the bead, it indicates potential decompensated exophoria.
- If the subject struggles to see the two strings clearly, even after wiggling the string, it suggests suppression in one eye, which can impact aiming ability.

The Brock string thus provides valuable insights into the binocular vision of athletes, aiding in the identification of potential visual anomalies that may affect their performance in sports.

Color Preference Test

The color preference test serves dual purposes—it assesses light sensitivity and provides insight into color preferences, aiding in the selection of appropriate tinting for prescriptions. For many athletes, the results of this test can be striking, prompting immediate inquiries about their significance and relevance.

In the context of sports, which are predominantly played outdoors, consideration must be given to the potentially damaging effects of strong sunlight, blue light, and ultraviolet radiation. Understanding an individual's

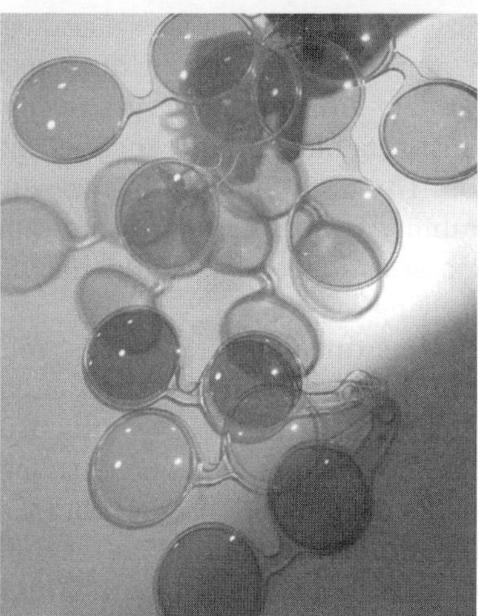

Fig. 6.2: Color preference test.

light sensitivity and color preferences becomes essential for estimating the appropriate level of tint required for their specific needs.

The color preference test **(Fig. 6.2)** not only helps identify the optimal tint for mitigating the effects of outdoor light but also enhances visual comfort and performance. By incorporating individual preferences and sensitivities into tint selection, athletes can better protect their eyes while optimizing their visual experience during sports activities.

ANALYTICAL TEST

Geraint also suggested that in sport vision assessment, there should be a test for specific visual skills that relate to the particular skills required in a given sport. These tests can be designed using skills recognized as crucial to individual sport. The advantage of such tests is that a group of athletes belonging to the same sport can be screened using the test, enabling a comparative analytical study of their performance to determine who requires a full eye examination. Since these tests are primarily intended for further analysis, Geraint proposed that they be called 'Analytical Tests.'

Analytical tests are pivotal in addressing the challenges athletes encounter in their chosen sports. Distinguished from diagnostic tests, they are sport-specific and serve as complex measures of visual performance within each respective sport. These tests allow for comparative assessments among athletes using skills recognized as critical to their individual sports, rather than being common across all sports.

Designed to impact at least two elements of visual skills listed in diagnostic tests, analytical tests transcend standard eye examinations. They exclusively evaluate visual abilities essential to overall athletic training and can also target the enhancement of specific visual skills. Moreover, they provide insights into how effectively athletes' visual system performs within their particular sports.

These tests may vary across different sports and can be designed by the optometrist based on their own knowledge of the respective sport or through discussions with the athlete. Analytical tests gauge complex visual functions that simulate crucial aspects of the sport, such as aiming, anticipation, or eye-hand coordination. The tests should prioritize simplicity, repeatability, and objective measurability. If an athlete consistently performs poorly on the analytical test, further assessment through other diagnostic tests is necessary to determine the underlying reasons.

In tennis, anticipation through depth judgment stands out as the predominant visual skill. Stereopsis tests can serve as effective analytical tools as they meet the criteria for such tests, being influenced by factors like poor visual acuity, particularly in one eye, and vergence function. A reduction in stereoscopic acuity may suggest potential issues with timing in shot execution.

The Bassin Anticipation Timer represents sophisticated equipment developed to assess anticipation via depth judgment and eye-hand coordination. The ability to accurately judge the distance and speed of approaching objects demands active accommodation, good vergence facility, visual acuity, and effective binocular coordination. This device simulates ball arrival through a sequence of diodes lighting up in succession. Athletes positioned at one end respond as soon as the nearest diode illuminates, mimicking the anticipation of a ball's trajectory. Delayed responses may indicate the presence of exophoria, which can be evaluated in clinical settings using tests like the Brock string or Howell Phoria tests.

Analytical tests can be as straightforward as ball catching, which evaluates an athlete's ability to catch a ball, relying on well-established eye dominance and strong depth perception, in addition to eye-hand coordination. In this test, the athlete is tasked with catching a ball thrown underarm from a distance of 20 feet. The number of successful catches is recorded against the number of missed catches for further analysis. The catcher utilizes their dominant eye to judge the ball's position in space and anticipates its arrival time using depth perception and visual cues like stereopsis. Consequently, this test proves effective in sports such as golf. However, some researchers argue that the act of catching a ball is often bolstered by an adrenaline surge during competitive events, potentially masking weaknesses in the binocular system, which is crucial for successful catching. While this argument may hold true in certain cases, the fundamental visual skill required for catching relies on good anticipation and a well-established dominant eye for consistent performance.

Dynamic Fixation test can also be good analytical test in sports that require eye movement as it fulfils the requirements of analytical tests to contain two or more elements of vision, i.e., vergence and accommodation facility. It also has its application in the measurement of eye speed and ability to change fixation quickly from point in space to another as seen in table tennis. Poor performance in Dynamic Fixation test may show poor vergence or focus facility that could affect anticipation timing. The time taken to change the focus from an object far away to near may affect reaction time and can cause to drop a pass or miss a hit or an easy volley.

Contrast sensitivity testing tool can also be used as analytical tests for day long sports where light level changes from time to time. Contrast sensitivity is important for judging the ball against a similar color background. Any deficit in this ability will make it difficult to see and follow the moving objects which could be the result of low contrast visual acuity and glare. It could also be effectively used in Fencing.

Dynamic Vision Rotator creates a visual simulation of dynamic visual acuity. It can be used as an analytical test in sports where it is critical to see the moving objects or vice versa or both the athletes and the objects are in motion. Deficits in this ability may be associated with deficits in visual acuity and depth perception.

Wayne Saccadic Fixator, Acuvision 1000, and Peripheral Awareness Test are some of the sophisticated equipment that can be used as analytical tests. Wayne Saccadic Fixator affects accommodation, vergence facility and saccadic eye movement and it can be good for sport where eye-hand coordination is the primary visual requirement. Acuvision 1000 can be effectively used as analytical tests in sports where eye-hand coordination is extremely important like boxing, hockey and fencing. Eye-hand coordination is the ability controls the hand movement guided by vision. It requires simultaneous use of eye and hand. Eye-hand coordination is a complex process that requires effortless visual performance in the areas of eye movements, focusing ability, eye teaming and peripheral awareness. Peripheral awareness test measures the visual ability of the athlete to be aware of peripheral objects while maintaining central vision. Deficits can cause the athlete to be distracted by the movement and objects in the peripheral field of vision.

Sports Vision Clinical Practice

7 CHAPTER

Once the preliminary diagnosis is established during the screening stage and the athlete agrees to undergo a complete clinical assessment, all standard eye examination procedures are conducted in a clinical setting. This includes tests such as the slit-lamp examination, fundus examination, and measurement of intraocular pressure.

Additionally, any tests performed during the initial screening may be repeated in the clinical setting for verification purposes. For instance, the Mallet tests can be used to validate the results obtained from the Brock string assessment. Prism correction can be effectively demonstrated using TNO tests, allowing for precise adjustments based on the athlete's visual needs.

Refraction, a critical measurement in sports vision assessment, is conducted with careful consideration of the visual requirements specific to the sport in question. This ensures that any corrective measures implemented are tailored to enhance the athlete's performance within their sporting environment.

By conducting thorough clinical assessments and repeating relevant tests as necessary, optometrists can precisely evaluate the athlete's visual health. This process lays the foundation for developing a strategy for further sport vision assessment, which may begin with a basic understanding of the athlete's sports and dominance profile.

Understanding the intricacies of the athlete's sport and dominance profile provides valuable insights into their visual needs and performance requirements. This initial assessment sets the stage for more targeted sport vision evaluations, enabling optometrists to tailor interventions and training programs to enhance the athlete's visual performance in their specific sporting context.

INITIATING THE PROCESS

In general, most clinical examination usually starts with history taking but for sport vision practice history taking may be kept on hold for second step as the practitioner already has basic information about athlete and his sporting performance collected during screening stage. Therefore, it is advisable to prioritize tests that serve as the cornerstone of the comprehensive sport vision examination. The three tests as shown in **Figure 7.1** may be considered to initiate the process.

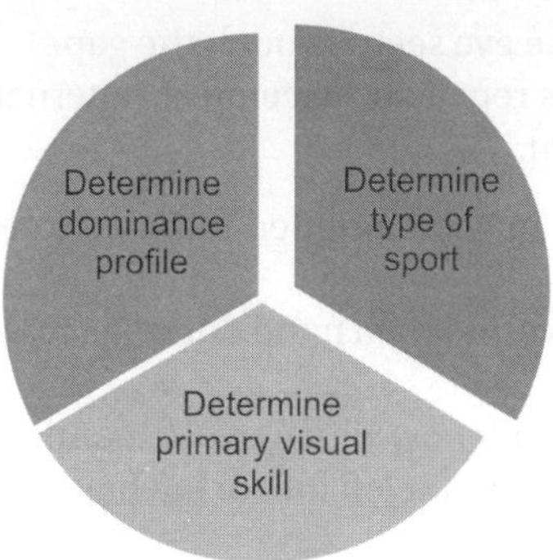

Fig. 7.1: Three tests to initiate the sport vision assessment.

Determine Dominance Profile

Although the eye dominance test has already been done during the screening, it is recommended to reassess eye dominance during the consulting room eye examination for the following reasons:

- Ocular dominance is crucial in understanding the relationship between vision and sporting performance.
- It influences decisions regarding correcting even minor refractive errors in binocular vision correction, especially in sports requiring precise aiming like darts, archery, and shooting.
- Eye dominance can predispose individuals to specific sports, and an incorrect configuration may hinder competitive performance.
- Understanding eye dominance is pivotal in addressing visual challenges in sports, as it is highly specific to each sport and can significantly impact athletic abilities.

The "Hand over hand method" is the preferred test for determining eye dominance in sport vision examinations. Geraint Griffiths, in his paper "Eye Dominance in Sport—A Comparative Study," highlights its significance. This method offers several advantages:

- By focusing on the observer's nose rather than one eye or the other, the test ensures symmetry in the assessment process.
- Alternating hands prevent bias towards the left or right side.
- Unlike the hole-in-the-card method, it minimizes the possibility of head movement to peek through the card hole.
- The method consistently produces results, even if there's occasional hesitation, which is important for accurate recording.

The process for determining eye dominance is as follows:

- Athlete places hands in front of them.
- Athlete places right hand over left, leaving a small gap between the apexes of the index finger and thumb.
- Athlete extends hands until the examiner's nose is visible through the gap.
- Examiner records the eye seen through the gap.
- Athlete places left hand over right, again leaving a small gap between the apexes of the index finger and thumb.

- Examiner records the eye seen through the gap.
- The measurement is repeated twice more, alternating between right over left and left over right.

The results of the tests may be grouped into two categories based on ocular dominance:

1. Athletes with right eye and right hand dominance, representing strong right dominance.
2. Athletes with a left tendency, which could manifest even subtly during the test either as a preference for left foot or left hand or left dominant response during dominant eye test.

Lateral dominance, observed in both physical and ocular aspects, illustrates how individuals favor one side of their body or ocular system for specific tasks or conditions. Dominance profiles include combinations such as:

- Dominant right eye and right hand
- Dominant left eye and left hand
- Dominant right eye and left hand
- Dominant left eye and right hand and so on

Understanding lateral dominance sheds light on how individuals process information and learn from their surroundings. It influences learning characteristics and behavior, particularly in stressful situations. Recognizing dominance profiles provides insights into an individual's strengths and challenges, aiding in the development of effective learning strategies. In sports vision practice, understanding the implications of eye dominance in binocular vision and its relation to hand and body dominance is essential **(Fig. 7.2).**

It is important to note that eye dominance is not always indicative of hand dominance, highlighting the need to assess hand dominance separately. Tasks such as scissor and paper cutting, as well as holding a pen, can be utilized to determine hand dominance accurately.

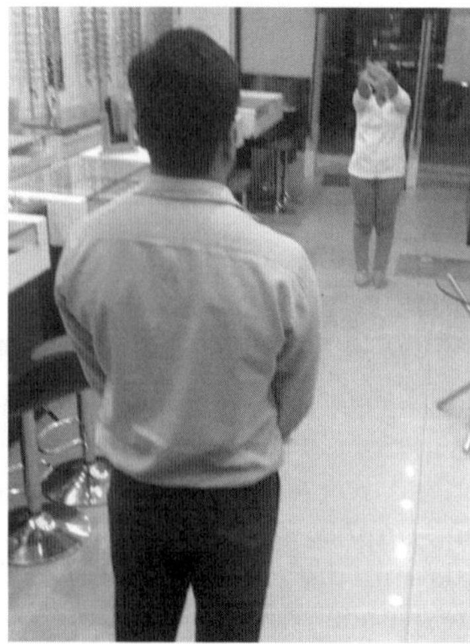

Fig. 7.2: Hand over hand method.

Determine Primary Visual Skill

The next is to assess the proportions of aiming and anticipation inherent to the athlete's chosen sport. Assessing the proportions of aiming and anticipation in an athlete's chosen sport is integral to sports vision examination. Each sport exhibits varying degrees of aiming and anticipation, which must be evaluated to understand the athlete's precise visual requirements.

Aiming entails positioning sights relative to the target, facilitating steady fixation, while anticipation enables athletes to gauge the speed and direction of moving objects for timely responses. Effective anticipation prevents mistiming, while aiming prevents misalignment. Establishing the primary visual need in each sport guides further sports vision investigation effectively.

Determine Type of Sport

Geraint proposed that sports can be categorized into two main types: Dynamic and Non-dynamic. *Dynamic sports* involve explosive movements, high speed, and quick actions, posing a greater risk of trauma. Examples include 100-meter running, football, and squash. *Non-dynamic sports,* on the other hand, feature slow, controlled, and repetitive actions that may span overextended periods. Consistency in performance is key, as seen in sports like chess and shooting.

While some sports may seem static, the mental demands in activities like chess and shooting are immense. Athletes must maintain precise control and spatial awareness, compensating for the lack of physical dynamism with intense mental effort. The line between dynamic and non-dynamic sports may blur, understanding these distinctions is crucial for applying sports vision principles effectively.

ROUTINE PROCEDURE

A series of routine tests are now conducted to thoroughly assess the vision and visual system, as depicted in **Figure 7.3**.

History Taking

In sports vision practice, history-taking transcends a mere checklist of symptoms; it serves as a pivotal platform for engaging in meaningful two-way communication. Employing a case-based discussion approach fosters a natural exchange of information, allowing athletes and practitioners to collaborate effectively. The history-taking process sets the stage for shared objectives among athletes, coaches, and practitioners, enhancing mutual understanding and cooperation. Key questions to establish goals include:

- Current use and experience with visual aids
- Lifestyle, medications, and dietary habits
- Sports participation, position, and role
- Recent changes in sporting performance
- Perception of any visual difficulties

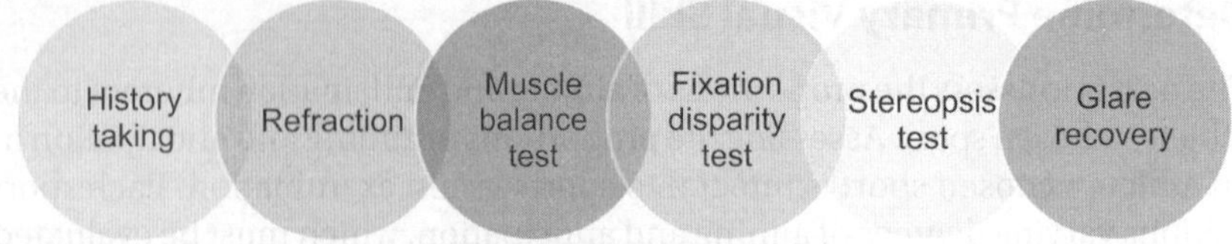

Fig. 7.3: Routine tests.

- Participation in vision training programs
- Identification of recurring difficulty areas
- Athlete's concerns regarding sporting performance

Refraction

Good refraction is indeed the cornerstone of optimal visual performance. Unless visual acuity is maximized during the refraction process, the subsequent steps in dispensing corrective measures lose their significance. This becomes especially critical when there is an intensified pressure of excessive visual demands on the visual system, such as those encountered in sports or other visually demanding activities. As a general rule, it is advisable to first prescribe for any significant refractive error because improper correction of refractive error:

- Result in either under or over-accommodation, resulting in disorders of accommodative functions. Such disorders can hinder an athlete's ability to focus on dynamic and rapidly changing visual stimuli, affecting their overall performance.
- Results in a high phoria and demands unusual negative or positive fusional vergence. This may affect an athlete's ability to maintain binocular vision and coordinate eye movements effectively, which is essential for activities requiring precision and accuracy.
- Creates an imbalance between the two eyes, leading to sensory fusion disturbances. Maintaining proper alignment and coordination is crucial for optimal visual performance, and disruptions can hinder an athlete's ability to perform at their best.
- Creates decreased fusional ability as a result of blurred retinal images. Reduced ability to fuse images can compromise an athlete's overall visual function, affecting their ability to process visual information accurately.

Even the small degree of refractive error may become significant for someone. Therefore, the practitioner must take this decision based on additional testing and analysis of accommodative and binocular vision function so that he can answer whether the refractive error is the cause of the poor visual performance. This involves a more nuanced and holistic approach to vision care.

Two Scenarios Generally Exist

First, the athlete may present with significant accommodative and binocular vision problems. In such a situation, the low refractive error becomes significant as it will improve fusion and assist in management.

Another possible situation may be a patient with low refractive error, and all the accommodative and binocular testing results are within expected values. In this case, the practitioner may be left with no other possible visual basis for the patient's discomfort and must make a decision about prescribing the low refractive error. Experience shows that there is often an accommodative, ocular motor, or binocular vision disorder present in addition to low refractive error. It is very unusual to find a low refractive error in isolation that accounts for significant symptoms.

All myopic refractive errors, even 0.50D should be considered for correction in sports. Correction of 0.50D or more of anisometropia should be contemplated, especially if it requires accurate depth perception. In addition, the effect of meridional anisometropia should be considered in athletes with asymmetric astigmatism. Correction of hypermetropia over 1.00D can alleviate fatigue, particularly in sports requiring sustained visual attention at the middle of the target. Astigmatism of more than 0.50D may reduce contrast and therefore should be considered. A young sport person with a little over minus correction will provide maximum distance visual acuity, albeit at the expense of having to exert a minor accommodative effort.

Once the full refraction is known, then refinements can be made, depending upon the visual need of the sport. A task analysis of the sport will assist in determining the specific visual demands and a careful refractive analysis can establish the best refractive compensation for use in that sport. For example, a myopic baseball player may be benefit from an additional 0.25D of minus to improve contrast when playing in twilight conditions. Billiards has specific viewing distances that should be considered, especially for presbyopic athletes. Billiard's players often use single vision intermediate distance prescription for use during play. In sports like tennis where near visual acuity has minimal impact on performance, prescription of near addition may be avoided. In Golf also near visual acuity doesn't affect performance, however clear vision is desirable for seeing the score card and identifying one's ball during the play. Such prescription becomes sports specific and is not prescribed for general use.

The toughest challenge for refractive error correction is created by shooters. Rifle shooters require that the shooters clearly focus the target at far distance while carefully aligning the front and rear sights of the rifle with the target. There are four things in this equation—the aiming eye, the rear sight, front sight, and the target. The participant peeps through the sights, and sees three circles. He has to align these circles concentrically with the target in the middle. It is very important to have a clear picture of the sights than the target in rifle shooting. Once the sight has stabilized, pressure must be applied to the trigger to release the shot.

Pistol shooters are particularly affected by presbyopia because the front and rear sights must be aligned with the target with extreme precision. Front sight is positioned at an intermediate distance from the eyes and the difference in accommodative demand between sights and the far target creates significant blur for one distance when focusing at the other. The pistol shooters often want solution that provides image clarity at both the distances. Pistol shooters need a clear picture of sight. They require more additional plus power than Rifle shooters. Younger shooters should be given little less near additional plus power so that they can also use the accommodation while keeping enough in reserve to avoid eye fatigue. The correction should be prescribed with an executive bifocal which will not induce image jump.

Consideration for Prescribing Correction

The following important consideration must be kept in mind while prescribing correction for athletes and players:

- Even the smallest amount of refractive error must be corrected. In visually demanding occupation like sports, small amount of uncorrected myopia affects the visual performance. The visual system detects the blur and is left with no other option but to accommodate which effectively make them more myopic.
- In case of uncorrected low astigmatism, the visual system is in flux looking for a point focus and potentially causing a degree of accommodative spasm which ultimately makes it more difficult to relax accommodation sufficiently.
- Care must be taken while doing refraction in amblyopic eye. Peripheral awareness in this eye can be as good as other eye and uncorrected hypermetropia may have effect on the other eye and muscle balance between the two eyes.
- In squinting eyes, the abnormal retinal correspondence will contribute to a degree of depth perception which may be enhanced by same consideration as above.
- Refinement is very critical in sports vision refraction. Once the subjective refraction is determined, it is important to provide allowance for the required distance. For example, in shooting the athletes already have good acuity. Leaving them with correction at 6 meters will not give them sufficient flexibility and control at greater distance. It should also be remembered that in competitive situation, huge level of adrenalin will give them additional energy to accommodation that may not be seen during consulting room examination.
- The oculomotor balance may be affected by refraction. Uncorrected hyperopia can induce decompensated esophoria. Under corrected myopia may force an athlete to go into overdrive searching for clear focus. The effect of over correction may be influenced by relationship between accommodation and vergence function which may vary from one person to another.

The mechanics of refraction applied is also extremely important, for example binocular balancing and accurate testing of fixation disparity should be routinely practiced in sport vision practice. Advice on refractive error cannot be given unless you know the dominant eye and which sport they particularly favor. This information is to be kept in mind throughout the whole procedure. Peripheral awareness which is maximized by using high curve lenses and contact lenses can also be affected by residual uncorrected refractive error which will tend to diminish visual performance and eventually will make the athlete less peripherally aware.

Muscle Balance Test

The way two eyes work together inevitably affect the ability of the visual system to judge distance and the position in the space. The coordinated use of six extra ocular muscles controlling the movement of each eye is indispensable to the restoration of good binocular vision. An assessment of muscle balance, therefore for distance and near vision is required to determine whether heterotropia or heterophoria is present or not. Cover Test, Maddox Rod test or Howell Phoria test can be used. Cover test is quick and useful but very often not as objective as the science requires. Howell Phoria is very fast and gives direction of the horizontal deviation and amount of prism diopter required to correct in one go. However, it's scope is limited to the convergence and divergence only. It cannot measure vertical deviations.

The Maddox Rod test is a diagnostic tool used in optometry to assess the presence and magnitude of ocular deviations, particularly phorias and tropias. It involves the use of a cylindrical lens with a red glass rod attached to one end. The patient views a distant target through the rod while one eye is covered, causing a horizontal red line to be superimposed over the visual field. The deviation of the line from a true horizontal position indicates the presence and direction of the deviation. In sport vision assessment, the Maddox Rod test can be valuable in detection of phorias and tropias which can affect an athlete's visual alignment, potentially impacting their performance in sports that require precise visual targeting, such as shooting or archery. It can also help assess how well the eyes work together to maintain alignment, which is crucial for depth perception and accurate judgment of distances, essential skills in sports like tennis, baseball, or golf. The Maddox Rod test can assess how ocular alignment changes in response to different lighting conditions, helping identify potential challenges athletes may face during competition.

Fixation Disparity Test

The muscle balance test has to be followed by Fixation disparity test to confirm that the muscle balance is leading to observable effects on eye coordination. Brock string test usually done during the screening gives lot of information about the visual system and provokes questions from the athletes and allows the practitioner to relate what they observe and their performance difficulties on the field of play. The similar test can be done in clinic with Mallet test. The two-string effect is equivalent to nonius bars within the black circle. Fixation disparity is measured separately for distance and near. It reduces level of stereopsis. The subject may have different level of fixation disparity at distance and near. Misalignment may be horizontal, vertical or both. Prism is needed to correct the fixation disparity.

Stereopsis Test

Stereopsis is measured with TNO test. The test consists of seven plates. First three plates, enable the examiner to quickly establish whether stereoscopic vision is present at all. Plate 4 is for the suppression test and then next three plates may be used for exact determination of stereoscopic acuity. When used for screening purpose, only plate 5 should be used as a pass-fail criterion. It is important to place the test at 40 cm with correction in place and squarely in front of the subject. Reduced stereopsis may indicate the presence of poor timing.

Glare Recovery Test

The glare recovery test is a crucial clinical assessment in sports vision practice, aiming to evaluate the impact of glare on visual function.

A functional approach to understand the effect of glare on eyes may be as under:

- Measuring visual acuity using a LogMAR chart under standard lighting conditions.
- Repeat the visual acuity measurement while shining a bright light from an ophthalmoscope or a torch directly into the subject's eyes.
- Note any decrease in visual acuity, typically indicated by a drop of one or two lines on the chart, signifying a significant effect of glare.

Glare recovery time holds significance in sports, as it reflects the speed at which the visual system restores function after exposure to bright light. Conditions or factors influencing light and dark adaptation can impact glare recovery, potentially predicting an individual's susceptibility to retinopathy. During the test, recovery time is measured in seconds required to regain visual acuity to the actual level following disability glare induced by a camera flash held at a distance of 2 or 3 meters.

ADDITIONAL TESTS

In sport vision clinical assessment, three additional tests are utilized to evaluate critical visual skills essential for peak sporting performance. These tests offer valuable insights into an athlete's visual abilities and aid in customizing training programs to improve specific skills required for their sport. They are explained below:

Eye-Hand Coordination

Eye-hand coordination is crucial, particularly in dynamic sports, where the rapid and accurate synchronization between visual input and motor response is paramount. Assessing the speed and precision of eye-hand coordination in response to visual stimuli is a key component of sport vision assessment, as it directly influences timing and reaction capabilities. Deficiencies in eye-hand coordination can hamper performance levels in eye-led sports such as cricket, boxing, and tennis by delaying the athlete's response time. Tools like the Acuvision 1000 and Bassin Anticipation Timer are utilized to evaluate eye-hand coordination effectively.

Dynamic Fixation Test

Dynamic Fixation test is used to measure the eye speed, i.e., to evaluate the athletic ability to change focus rapidly and smoothly while looking from distance to near and back again. It measures the muscle's speed which is interesting, because it is entirely dependent on the speed of extra ocular muscles. This in turn is important in sport, because that is where locomotion comes from. The time taken to complete a cycle is recorded three times with the help of stopwatch. Poor performance on the Dynamic Fixation test may indicate deficiencies in vergence or focus facility, potentially affecting anticipation timing. Slow focus transitions from far to near could impact reaction time, leading to missed passes or volley opportunities.

Anticipation Test

Bassin Anticipation Timer can be used to assess anticipation timing. Using this instrument, the athlete may respond early, i.e., may press the button to stop the light too early. The convention is to label this as a "negative value". Sometimes he may press the button too late. A late response is given a positive value. He may press the button too late or too early in a random fashion indicating that their judgment of anticipation is generally inaccurate. The measure of inaccuracy is given by the spread of the results. Ten trials are done and then a mean response in milliseconds of the ten results is derived to actually define whether the athlete is responding early or late. A late response seems to be the norm, i.e., letting the ball come on the bat, avoiding getting under the ball. For a single elite group, the comparative data for each member of that group is very useful to predict which of the players is suffering a visual deficit. Late anticipation may correspond to exophoria on Brock string test. Poor timing on basin is associated with reduced depth judgment and vice versa.

More tests and techniques can be employed on a case-by-case basis during assessment in optometry. Optometrists should be prepared to apply them as necessary and base their diagnosis on the results of the entire battery of tests, rather than relying solely on one or two assessments. Once the diagnosis is established in the consultation room using comprehensive tests, optometrists can effectively provide a visual explanation of the athlete's sporting difficulties. This approach may help restore the lost confidence of the athlete. Some of the examples are tabulated as examples in **Table 7.1**.

The immediate practical implications underscore that in numerous sports, vision often stands as the single most significant barrier to enhancing performance. It is likely to be the foremost consideration in preparing for competitive sports. Enhancing vision does not automatically make a great athlete; rather, it removes a barrier to improving athlete performance,

Table 7.1: Examples of how to explain an athlete's sporting deficiency in relation to visual factors.

Sporting deficiency	*Probable associated visual factor*	*Probable solution*
Missing the target to the left of gold in archery	Left nondominant eye taking over	Restore right dominant eye with full correction
Late breaking and too much speed going into the corner while right hand bends in car racing	Convergence insufficiency makes track markers appear further away than they are. A left medial rectus paresis may be the reason for right hand bends	Orthoptic exercise may help
Fair skin, light blue eye player feeling disability during bright sunny day in soccer	Light sensitivity	Tinted contact lenses may help
Goalkeeper losing confidence in catching high balls or going down to the feet of oncoming players	Incipient myopia and astigmatism causing accommodative spasm with an associated decompensated esophoria	Correction of myopia and astigmatism may help to look at the situation

allowing them to compete on more equal terms. It's probable that exceptional athletes in highly visual sports possess superior vision; achieving such levels of performance would likely be unattainable without it.

Therefore, managers bear the responsibility of ensuring that teams undergo regular vision screenings. It is a common observation among eye care practitioners that many individuals, including athletes, are unaware of underperforming vision. Regular screening is essential for all athletes, not only to enlighten them about the visual process but also to ensure they have no deficiencies. Even the slightest degree of blur in just one eye can significantly impair the ability to hit a target or score goals.

Sports Vision Therapy

8 CHAPTER

A thorough examination of every facet of visual skills is essential before embarking on specialized sports vision therapy. These assessments must be conducted meticulously, aligning them with the specific visual requirements of the athlete's chosen sport. It's crucial to conduct the assessment in a manner that allows for the detection of even the most subtle defects in visual skill.

Moreover, the assessment should be designed to identify any compensatory mechanisms that the athlete may be employing to compensate for deficiencies in visual skills. Athletes often sacrifice other abilities to cope with increasing cognitive and physical loads, highlighting the importance of uncovering such compensations during the evaluation process.

Once the assessment is complete, the results should be recorded and compared against both the ideal levels of visual skills and the visual abilities of peers competing at the same level in the sport. This comparative analysis forms the basis for devising a tailored therapy plan aimed at enhancing visual skills and ensuring their seamless integration with other athletic abilities.

In sports vision therapy, activities are selected and sequenced to refine existing visual behaviors, promoting greater efficiency and precision. Athletes are encouraged to practice these selected activities both in clinical settings and at home, gradually increasing the level of challenge until the desired visual behaviors become automatic and sustained. Ultimately, the goal is to equip athletes with visual skills that can meet the demands of their sport effectively.

TRAITS OF SPORTS VISION THERAPY

The sports vision therapy should have following attributes:

- Sports vision therapy must align with the athlete's specific sport and position to maximize motivation and participation. Athletes are driven by performance-oriented activities tailored to their sport, seeking justification and objective progress monitoring for each task.
- Athletes rely on precise timing and movement coordination to navigate space effectively and assume optimal positions. Therefore, sports vision therapy activities should focus on integrating visual skills like eye movements and hand-eye coordination with timing, facilitating seamless movement and positioning.
- Elite athletes often rely on swift and precise visually directed reactions, a crucial aspect of high-level sports performance. Sports vision therapy activities are designed to enhance this capability by emphasizing and providing feedback on the speed of accommodative or vergence responses,

as well as eye-hand coordination skills. By focusing on these elements, athletes can develop the rapid reaction abilities necessary for success at the elite level.

- In various sports, the predominant direction of gaze is specific to the athlete's position and the requirements of the chosen sport. This specificity underscores the need for tailored sports vision therapy interventions. For instance, certain sports demand superior gaze for optimal performance, such as baseball outfielders tracking flying balls, volleyball players anticipating overhead serves, or basketball power forwards assessing incoming plays. Conversely, some sports may require more frequent use of lateral or downward gaze depending on positional demands. Despite the importance of superior gaze in these scenarios, it's noteworthy that up gaze is not the natural visual direction for most individuals. Therefore, sports vision therapy interventions in such cases should prioritize the development of high-quality and sustainable binocular fusion and stereopsis in upward gaze positions. This targeted approach ensures athletes can effectively adapt their visual skills to the specific demands of their sport, enhancing performance and minimizing errors.
- In sports, body posture is rarely upright and is almost always dynamic, necessitating correct alignment for optimal performance. Efficient posture enables athletes to move swiftly and conserve energy, while inefficient posture requires more effort and time to compensate for poor alignment. Sports vision therapy plays a crucial role in enhancing visual skills across various postures. Postural dynamics directly impact gaze direction and eye movements, highlighting the need for tailored interventions. For example, wrestlers must maintain precise eye movements even in unconventional postures, while basketball players must exhibit visual efficiency in lateral gaze positions during hitting. Given the significance of body posture in sports, therapy programs should be designed with careful consideration of postural dynamics. By addressing visual skills in tandem with body alignment, athletes can optimize their performance, react effectively to dynamic situations, and minimize the energy expenditure associated with inefficient movement patterns.
- Once the visual skills are developed to appropriate levels in static situation, the athletes should be asked to practice on balance board, walking rails, rebounder or hopping while practicing visual skills like tracking or accommodation. This integration is important to translate clinical visual performance into field visual performance.
- Sports vision therapy activities should also consider the factors like lighting condition and noise so that visual performance can be maintained under expected visual environment.

TOOLS AND THERAPIES

Several sports vision therapies can be used to develop visual performance in sports. A basic knowledge of different therapies in relation to specific visual skills is helpful in designing appropriate sports vison therapy program for an athlete.

Visual Acuity

Static visual acuity and contrast sensitive function should be maximized with appropriate correction either with spectacle or with contact lenses and right tint selection. Dynamic visual acuity improves with training. However, in clinic a rotator chart or static visual acuity chart with the athlete in motion on a balance board or rebounder can be used.

Accommodation–Vergence Function

Accommodation and vergence constitute a reciprocal neurological system crucial for visual function. Enhancing accommodation accuracy, facility, and integration with vergence is achievable through targeted sports vision therapy. This allows athletes to swiftly and accurately shift focus between targets, promoting sustainability in performance. Techniques such as Loose Lens Rock, Mental Minus, Bifocal Rock, and Flippers are highly effective activities. They provide excellent subject's feedback to learn what it feels like to focus near or far and to develop fine control of accommodation in space.

Binocular Vision

The primary goal of binocular vision therapy is to cultivate stable, accurate, and adaptable vergence function. Minimal phoria across all gaze directions is imperative. Convergence and divergence should exhibit swift and automatic transitions between near and far targets. Monocular inequality should be absent, with efficient binocularity maintained across all gaze directions. Fusion must remain stable across varying distances and gaze directions, devoid of significant suppression. Stereo sensitivity should be optimized, with rapid and uniform performance across all gazes. Therapy tools such as the Brock string, prism flippers, vectograms, and stereo activities prove instrumental in achieving these objectives.

Eye Movements

The therapeutic aim is to enhance spontaneous, rapid, and precise pursuits and saccades across all gaze directions and body postures, ensuring resilience amidst movement and changes in balance. Utilizing tools like the Hart chart, Marsden ball, and dynamic fixation charts facilitates this improvement process.

Eye-Hand-Body Coordination

The core goal of sports vision therapy is to cultivate rapid and precise eye-hand and eye-foot coordination. Integrating tools like the Wayne Saccadic

Fixator or Acuvision 1000 into therapy regimens is highly beneficial. These tools not only offer targeted therapies but also provide built-in feedback and motivation for athletes through performance scores.

Central-Peripheral Awareness

Peripheral vision plays a crucial role in responding to the total spatial volume of the visual environment, particularly in sports contexts. Its significance lies not only in receiving information but also in the response it triggers. Serving as an early warning system, peripheral vision guides movement responses effectively. Therapeutic tools such as the Wayne Saccadic Fixator, Acuvision 1000, Walking rail, and Yoked prism are instrumental in enhancing central peripheral awareness. Moreover, plus lenses enhance peripheral awareness by blurring details and emphasizing the periphery, while minus lenses reduce visual space and accentuate central vision.

APPROACH TO THERAPY ACTIVITIES

The first step in designing a sports vision therapy program involves prescribing refractive correction through spectacles or contact lenses, especially if the correction is to be utilized during competitions. Even minor refractive errors can significantly impact visual performance. In some instances, solely correcting refractive errors may suffice to enhance visual capabilities. When sports vision therapy is recommended, optometrists should oversee progress through regular performance evaluations, typically occurring every 4 to 6 weeks.

Monocular skills, encompassing input, processing, and output, should be honed and balanced. Therapeutic interventions should facilitate equal ease and speed across monocular abilities including accommodation, pursuits, saccades, directional sense, and information processing. Practice sessions should continue until newly acquired visual skills become automatic while maintaining peripheral awareness.

Subsequently, binocular therapy should be initiated; gradually increasing the workload until efficient and accurate input, processing, and output are achieved. Augmenting the load may involve introducing movement, balance challenges, varying gaze factors, and altering bodily postures. Stressors such as timing constraints, environmental noise, and fluctuating lighting conditions should be incorporated to bolster visual skills' resilience under competitive pressures commonly encountered in sports.

Athletes may also be asked to practice therapy while talking because the athlete may be required to process visual information simultaneously with auditory information in certain sports. Calls from teammates for a pass or warning should be recognized without detracting from visual intake and visuomotor action.

Sports Vision Dispensing

9 CHAPTER

Dispensing represents the art of translating clinical assessments into practical visual solutions. It holds particular significance in sports, where optimal visual performance is intricately tied to athletic achievement. As a specialized field within ophthalmic optics, the primary aim of dispensing is to maximize the conveyance of visual information.

In the realm of sports, where split-second decisions and precise movements define success, the role of dispensing becomes even more critical. Any hindrance to the seamless transmission of visual cues can significantly impact an athlete's performance. Therefore, it is imperative that dispensing occurs in tandem with the initial clinical assessments, ensuring a coherent continuum of care.

A meticulous refraction and binocular balance, essential components of the clinical evaluation process, stand incomplete without proper dispensing. The alignment between clinical insights and practical implementation is key to unlocking an athlete's visual potential and enhancing overall performance. **Figure 9.1** illustrates the three primary modes of vision correction utilized to translate clinical findings into practical outcomes.

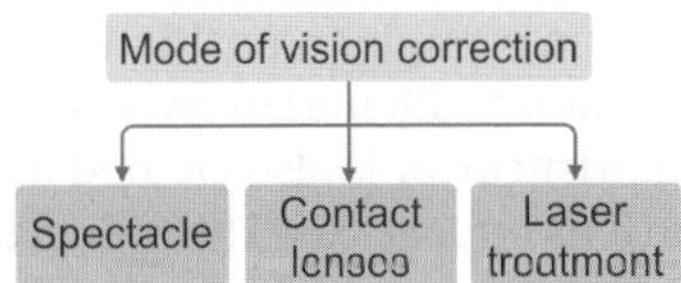

Fig. 9.1: Three modes of vision correction.

SPECTACLES

Spectacles, commonly known as eyeglasses, are optical devices worn in front of the eyes primarily to correct refractive errors and improve vision. They consist of lenses mounted in a frame that rests on the bridge of the nose and ears. Apart from vision correction, spectacles are also used as safety glasses, fashion accessories, and, in some cases, to enhance visual performance in specialized activities like sports or computer use. Thus, there are two main components of spectacles: frames and lenses.

Frames are the structures that hold the lenses in place and provide support for the spectacles. They come in various styles, materials, and designs, each offering different benefits and aesthetic appeal. Broadly, there are two types of frames: Regular frames or dress wear frames and sports frames or wrap frames.

Lenses are the optical components of spectacles that correct vision by focusing light appropriately onto the retina. They come in different types based on the specific vision correction needed and can be made from various materials. Like sports frames, there are specially designed sports lenses. We will restrict our discussion to sports frames and sports lens only.

Sports Frames

Sports frames as the means for carrying the lenses are critical in sports vision dispensing. Along with light level, rain, mist, and environmental factors, the position of the frame also has an impact on visual performance. Sports frames are not flat across the front. They are designed to have a wrap construction that follows the curvature of the face. They are either full-rimmed or supras. The wrap-shaped frames have a larger "A" measurement than "B" measurement and fit closer to the eyes compared to dress-wear frames. Some sports frames may have straps that pass behind the head instead of conventional sides. The wrap design of sports frames demonstrates unique features when fitted to the face (**Table 9.1**).

In the new wrap configuration, the wearer is looking through the lens on a different optical axis corresponding to the wrapped positioning. Increased Pantoscopic Angle tilts the lens around the horizontal axis that results in power error and astigmatic error across the entire lens surface. Increased Panoramic Angle tilts the lens along the vertical axis and creates asymmetry between the nasal and temporal sides of the lens, resulting in power error and astigmatic error across the entire lens surface. The effect of tilt around the horizontal axis and vertical axis changes the effect of the lens for central and peripheral power. The frame occupies a position such that the center of the pupil lies appr 4 to 5 mm above the horizontal center line, resulting in base down prism. Horizontal prism error is also created due to the angle between the line of vision and the lens optical axis. The reduced vertex distance allows the lens to move towards the eyes which implies that refracted distance is greater than the fitted distance. The effect of reduced vertex distance also alters the effective lens prescription that needs to be compensated using Effective Lens Power Formula. The other common traits of sports frames are shown in **Figure 9.2**.

Table 9.1: Sports frames features as shown on face.

	Wrap sports frame	*Dress wear frame*
Average panoramic angle	15 to 20 degree	5 degree
Average pantoscopic angle	7 to 9 degree	3 to 5 degree
Average vertex fitting distance	11 mm	14 mm

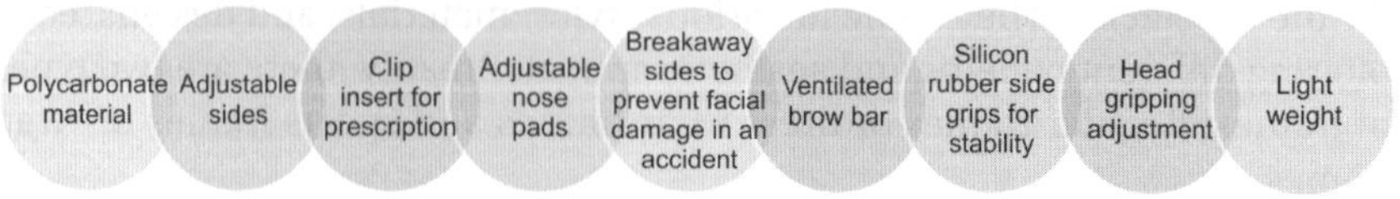

Fig. 9.2: Traits of sports frames.

Table 9.2: Advantages and disadvantages of using sports frames.

Advantages	*Disadvantages*
Safety from impact	Oblique astigmatism
Protection from side radiation and traumas	Unwanted prismatic effect
Protection from particles, pollen and wind	Different dioptric power
Complete UV protections	Leads to induce decentration
Possibility of wider peripheral vision	Impaired optical properties in the periphery
Decreased backside reflections	
Fashion statement	

The advantages and disadvantages of using sports frames are shown in **Table 9.2**.

Dihedral Angle

The horizontal inclination, also known as dihedral angle is the important differentiator when we compare sports frames with dress wear frames. Therefore, measuring dihedral angle is very critical. While measuring dihedral angle **(Fig. 9.3)**, the frame must be positioned on the head of the athlete because as the frame passes over the temples, it tends to decrease the horizontal inclination and hence measurements must be made in this situation. Dihedral angle is measured with frames using a specified tool for it. In addition, bridge size and eye shape are other two important measurements for dispensing sports frames.

Sports Lenses

Sports frames are uniquely designed with a wrap construction, contrasting starkly with dress wear frames in terms of face fit configurations. This wrap construction aids in shielding the eyes from side incident radiation, dust, pollen, and trauma, offering enhanced protection during athletic activities. However, fitting lenses into these sports frames presents distinct

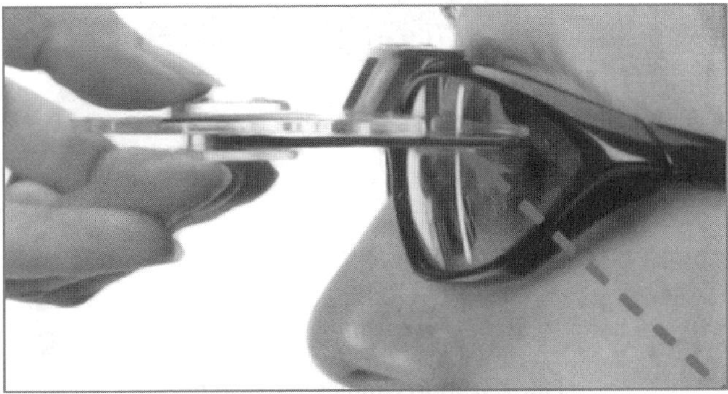

Fig. 9.3: Measuring dihedral angle.

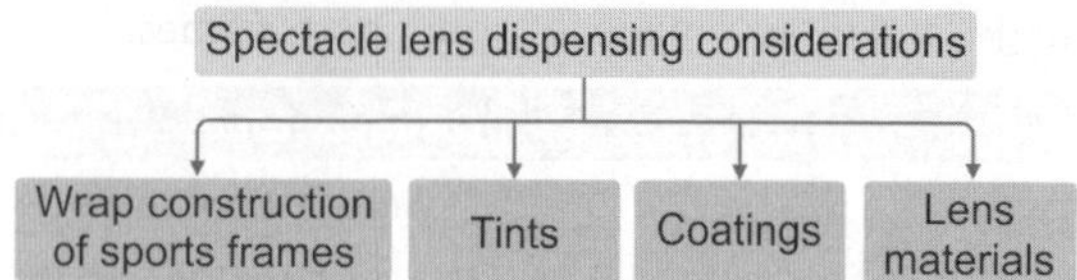

Fig. 9.4: Dispensing consideration for sports lens.

challenges that can be mitigated through the utilization of high base curve lenses. Moreover, there are additional considerations pertaining to vision enhancement and maintenance in the realm of sports eyewear. These specialized considerations are essential for dispensing spectacle lenses optimized for athletic performance, as mentioned in **Figure 9.4**.

SPECIALTY APPLIANCES

Specialty appliances for sports sunglasses are designed to optimize performance, comfort, and protection for athletes across a diverse range of sports and activities, the common among them are illustrated below:

Sports Frames with Clip (Fig. 9.5)

Sports frames may also be constructed with an insert clipped inside into which prescription lenses can be fitted. It may be with wrap or without wrap construction. This gets over the difficulties of the large eye size of sports frames. However, it creates the problem of two layers of lenses for the light to pass through. It means that there is a possibility of increased reflection and reduced light transmission. But it is a very useful option and with good coating these disadvantages can be minimized.

Swimming Goggle

Swimming goggles are cup-type lenses ensuring an eye seal, designed for surface swimming used to protect the eyes from chemical conjunctivitis and water borne microbes. They are available with prescription and without

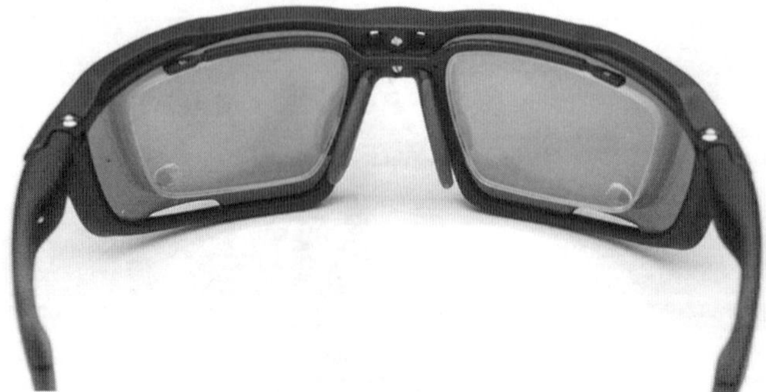

Fig. 9.5: Sports frames with clip on.

prescription and facilitate judgment of turns and direction as a vision correction tool **(Fig. 9.6)**.

Billiards Spectacles (Fig. 9.7)

Billiards needs high-fitting frames with joints at center or below to allow for low head position and relative up gaze.

Skiing Goggle (Fig. 9.8)

The skiing goggle needs to protect the eyes from trauma and ultraviolet radiations. It has to be well ventilated to maximize vision which may be the matter of life and death.

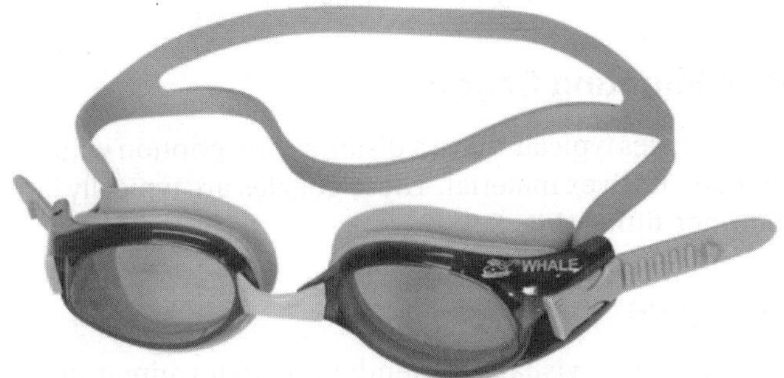

Fig. 9.6: Swimming goggle.

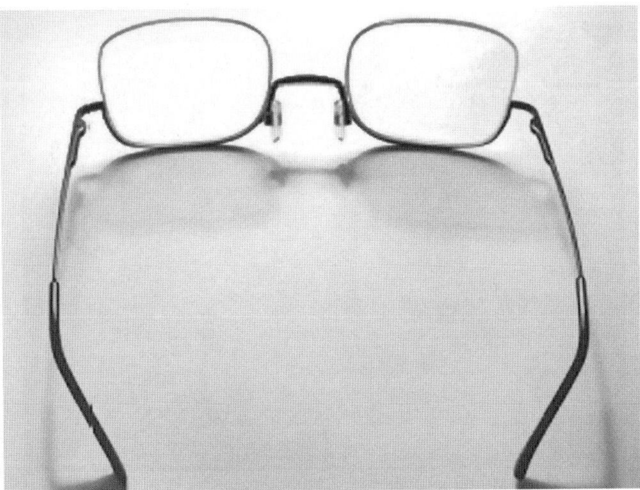

Fig. 9.7: Billiards spectacle.

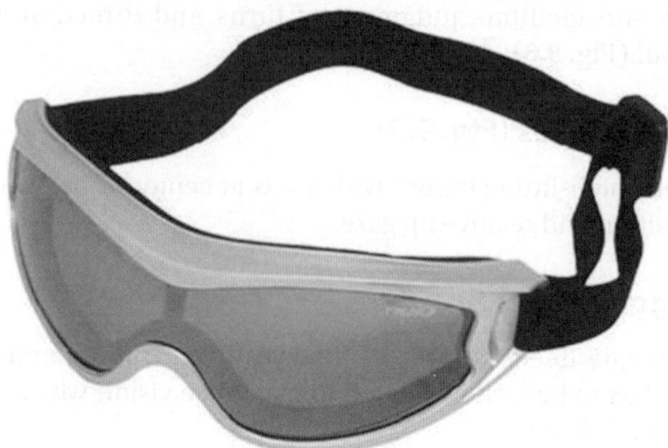

Fig. 9.8: Skiing goggle.

Clay Pigeon Shooting Goggle

Clay shooter's goggles typically have a distance prescription with lenses made of polycarbonate or trivex material. These goggles are typically large eye size with a high bridge fitting **(Fig. 9.9)**.

Shooting Goggle

Rifle shooting is highly visually dependent as determined by the angular substance of the target at the eye. The goggle provides precise correction in the aiming eye and occlusion of non-aiming eye, if needed **(Fig. 9.10)**.

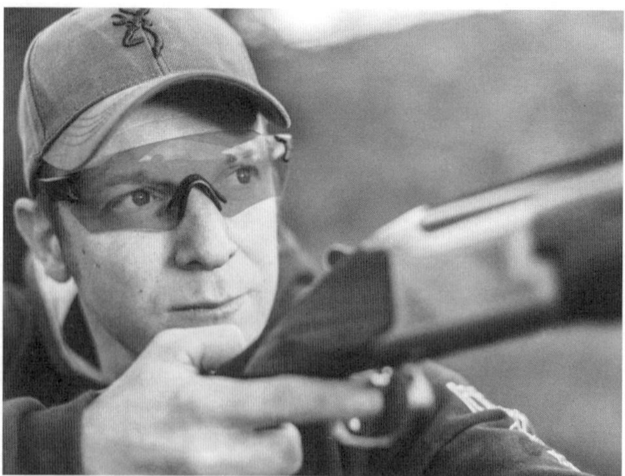

Fig. 9.9: Clay pigeon shooting goggle.

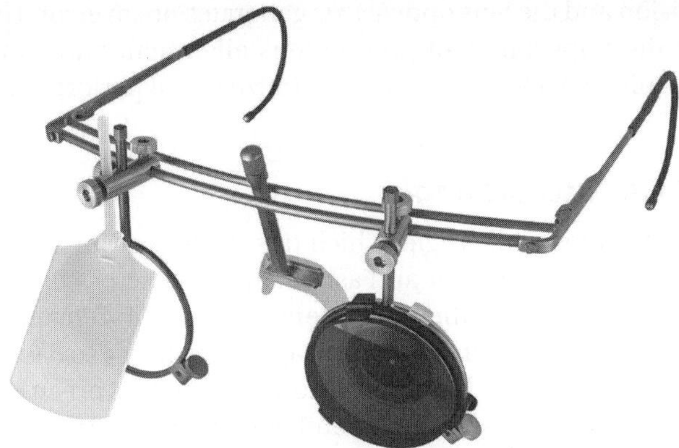

Fig. 9.10: Shooting goggle.

Wrap Construction of Sports Frames

The wrap construction of sports frames necessitates the fitting of high base curve lenses to maintain the streamlined appearance of the frames. For instance, inserting a -3.00 Dsph into an 8-base wrap frame requires surfacing it on an 8-base curve to uphold the appropriate lens fit. However, employing higher base curve lenses results in increased vertex distance and magnification of the wearer's visual field, leading to potential visual difficulties and dissatisfaction, particularly exacerbated by the degree of the wrap angle. This effect is elucidated in **Figure 9.11**, which illustrates the impact of high curved lenses on vision.

The disparity arises because the visual axis does not align with the optical axis of the lens. Consequently, the wearer perceives unwanted prism, oblique astigmatism, and blur due to the shifted optical axis caused by the wrapped positioning of the lens.

Addressing these challenges necessitates compensatory lens prescriptions to recalibrate the new lens prescription on both the X and Y axes, thereby improving visual clarity along the Z-axis and ensuring optimal vision at all viewing angles, including the periphery of the lens.

Increased Panoramic Angle

The increased panoramic angle inherent in high base curve lenses tilts the lens along the vertical axis, introducing asymmetry between the nasal and temporal sides of the lens. This asymmetry manifests as power error and

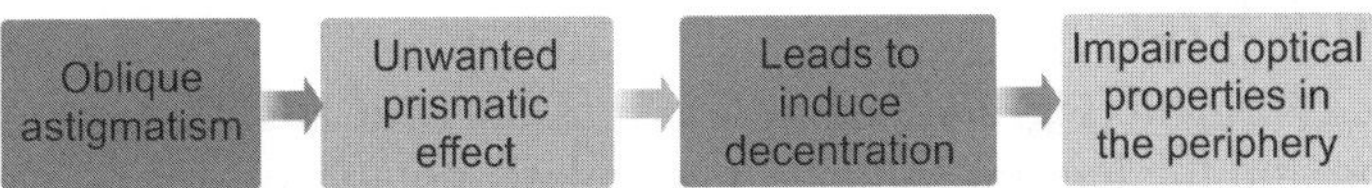

Fig. 9.11: Impact of high curved lenses on vision.

astigmatic error across the entire lens surface. Additionally, the angle between the line of vision and the lens optical axis generates prism error. These factors underscore the importance of precise lens alignment and compensation strategies to mitigate aberrations and optimize visual performance in sports eyewear.

Increased Pantoscopic Angle

The increased Pantoscopic Angle, which tilts the lens around the horizontal axis, contributes to power error and astigmatic error across the lens surface. This misalignment affects the entire lens surface. Moreover, the frame's positioning places the center of the pupil approximately 4 to 5 mm above the horizontal center line, introducing base down prism. This prism effect further complicates vision, necessitating careful consideration and adjustment to ensure optimal visual performance and comfort for the wearer.

Vertex Distance

In many wrap configurations of sports frames, the lens moves closer to the eyes, resulting in a refracted distance that exceeds the fitted distance. This alteration in vertex distance induces a change in the effective lens power, which can be calculated using the Effective Lens Power Formula. However, one significant limitation of dispensing measurements is the challenge of accurately measuring the vertex distance, particularly in the case of sports frames. The unique design and curvature of these frames make it difficult to obtain precise vertex distance measurements, complicating the accurate determination of effective lens power and potentially impacting visual correction outcomes.

Power Error

In a high wrap frame, the lens power undergoes rotation around two primary optical meridians—the tangential meridian, which lies along the horizontal plane, and the sagittal meridian, which revolves around the vertical plane. This rotational effect is commonly referred to as radial astigmatism, where the sagittal meridian represents the lens's spherical component, and the tangential meridian corresponds to the cylinder component.

The degree of the frame's wrap angle directly influences the amount of compensating lens power required. This holds true not only for sphero-cylindrical lenses but also for spherical lens powers. Additionally, the reduction in vertex distance caused by the frame's design further impacts the lens prescription, necessitating careful adjustment to ensure accurate visual correction and optimal vision quality for the wearer.

Prismatic Error

The Face Form tilt **(Fig. 9.12)** of the lens introduces an angle between the line of vision and the lens optical axis, particularly notable during convergence when the eyes are drawn inward. To counteract this effect, a relieving base in

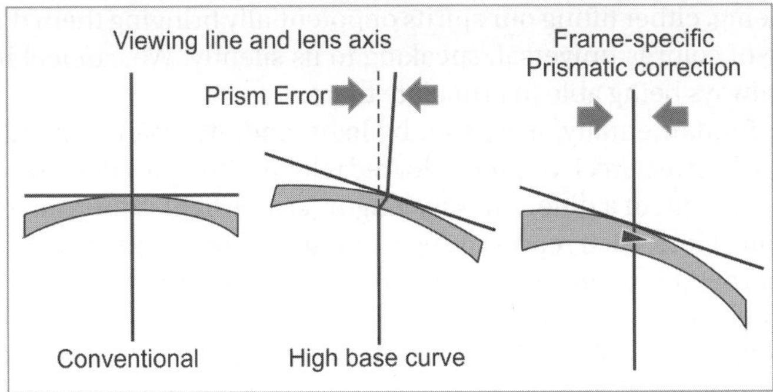

Fig. 9.12: Prismatic error.

prism is necessary. The magnitude of induced prism is influenced by several factors, as depicted in **Figure 9.13**.

The direction of the base of induced prism hinges on the point at which light enters the lens relative to the optical axis. In wrap-around frames, which inherently exhibit a greater degree of pantoscopic tilt, light typically enters the lens closer to the top, resulting in base-down prism. To offset this, a compensating lens must incorporate a neutralizing base-up prism component to ensure proper alignment and minimize visual distortion for the wearer.

The preparation of lenses that compensate for the aforementioned errors necessitates recalculations of lens power, resulting in what are commonly referred to as sports lenses. When dispensing sports lenses, it is crucial to take the following dispensing measurements into consideration to ensure optimal fit and visual correction for the wearer.

- Dihedral angle
- Pantoscopic angle
- Frame shape
- Bridge size
- Base curve
- Monocular PD
- Refractive error
- Refractive index of lens material
- Centre thickness of lens
- Diameter

Tints and Colors

Color communicates with us on a profound level, unlocking doors to our mind and spirit. It has the power to significantly impact our mood and overall sense

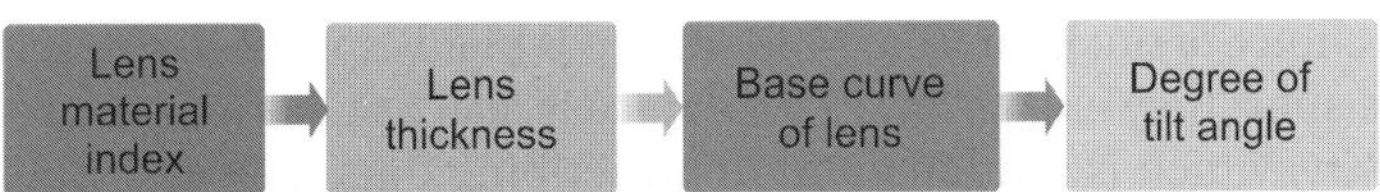

Fig. 9.13: Factors affecting induced prism.

of well-being, either lifting our spirits or potentially bringing them down. The language of color is universal, speaking to us silently. We can feel its effects without always being able to articulate them.

Color, fundamentally, is carried by light, and, in essence, it is light. For instance, what we perceive as the color red is light with a particular wavelength, while blue is light of a different wavelength. Visible light is the amalgamation of different colors, each representing a unique energy frequency. This energy can be harnessed to address health and behavioral issues stemming from subtle imbalances within the body.

The color of the objects that we see is largely due to the way those objects interact with light and ultimately reflect or transmit it to our eyes. We know that the visible light spectrum consists of a range of wavelengths that corresponds to a specific color. When visible light strikes an object and a specific wavelength is absorbed, that wavelength of light will not make it to our eyes. Any visible light that strikes the object and becomes reflected or transmitted to our eyes will contribute to the color appearance of the object.

For example, a green lens looks green because it absorbs all wavelengths except for those associated with green. Lenses are tinted simply to absorb light so that transmission is reduced. If all wavelengths of light are equally absorbed, it produces neutral gray, and if the absorption is different for different wavelengths, it produces a specific lens tint.

Therefore, the importance of tints in terms of protection and specific requirements cannot be underestimated in sports. The object of dispensing is to maximize vision. An athlete shouldn't solely decide how their lenses should be tinted; it cannot be left to their own choice. Even sunglasses should not be chosen without an optometrist's advice. The choice of tint is person-specific. A light-sensitive person may be reluctant to use yellow, while they may benefit from the use of blue.

Yellow is mostly used in shooting as it has a contrast-enhancing effect. Yellow absorbs blue and UV ends of the spectrum, which contribute to the veiling effect inside the globe, reducing contrast sensitivity. Blue light is focused in front of the retina, making it difficult to see, and UV radiation causes the optical media to fluoresce. Thus, someone who is not light-sensitive may report a dramatic improvement in clarity when using bright UV-filtering lenses like orange.

The older eyes with vitreous and crystalline lens opacities will tend to become more light sensitive because of light scattering effect, even if they were not naturally light sensitive.

When prescribing the blue tint for outdoor use, it should be noted that blue light carries the greatest amount of energy within each photon of light, so it is better to prescribe bluish-gray or bluish-green tints for outdoors which also have UV absorption.

The choice of tint is far from random and is highly specific to the individual and the sport they engage in. Color choice is also used as a measure of light sensitivity, which is fundamental to prescribing tints. The tint preferred in clinical tests is the summation of psychological as well as physical properties. Commonly, LT 80% is the first choice for indoors, and LT 20% for sun. The prescription of tint should be based on clinical decision. However, considering the environmental conditions needed for different sports, a general guideline can be worked upon what tints have been seen to be most effective in different sports.

Violet

Violet lies at shorter wavelength range of the visible spectrum. It is usually the least chosen color due to possibility of glare and the darkening effect. Even the light sensitive people refrain from violet preference.

Blue

Blue also lies at the shorter wavelength end of visible spectrum. The absorption in the yellow wavelength end makes it a good choice for light sensitive individuals. However, if there is a strong preference for blue, the prescription of blue for outdoor use should be avoided for:

- The danger of high energy blue light intensified by the brilliance of the sun.
- Likely to transmit more dangerous UV.
- The darkening effect of blue would allow pupil to dilate and increase exposure.

Note: Blue or bluish-gray tint is good for scuba diving, swimming.

Yellow

Yellow tint absorbs blue, violet and UV while allowing the transmission of a larger percentage of other wavelengths through. Yellow lies at the peak spectral acuity and hence concentrates light in the area of the spectrum to which the eye is most sensitive. If a person is already light sensitive, then the experience is heightened looking through yellow tint. Therefore, someone who is not light sensitive would surely appreciate contrast enhancing element of it especially during fading light condition. It is a good tint for shooting, snow skiing, hunting and tennis. A preference to yellow implies no light sensitivity and demand for high visual acuity.

Green

Green also lies near peak spectral acuity close to yellow. It has a good UV and blue light absorption and also has good infrared heat absorbing properties. This combination maximizes visual information while providing necessary protection. It also provides true color perception and protection from bright light. It is also contrast enhancer. It provides true color Perception. It makes a very good sunglass tint, because of its contrast enhancing properties and good UV absorption and heat protection. Golfers rely heavily on green filter to distinguish the ball from green ground. A preference to green implies light sensitivity and clouding of media.

Pink

Pink/Red has been found to be useful in hue discrimination in color deficient and migraine sufferers. It might be the color of choice in neurological patients. Pink has bright feel, usually favored by non-light sensitive persons and is a good UV and blue light absorber. It helps block blue light thereby improving contrast and offers high contrast and very soothing to the eyes. Many people feel that pink lenses are more comfortable for long periods of time than other lenses.

Brown

Optical brown is probably the best tint to protect the eye from UV and blue light and gives good comfort to light sensitive persons. It is a good tint for day driving. It also enhances contrast.

Orange

Orange is the essence of brown, so a tint diagnosis of orange would translate to brown tint. Using clinical judgments, this would be given indoors or outdoors at appropriate transmission level. Orange is the most commonly used tint for clay shooting. They are good to enhance visual performance and comfort. A preference to orange implies less light sensitivity and clouding of media.

Gray

Gray is a neutral density filter which does not distort color. Gray is the general purpose tint because it tames bright sunlight. It is likely to be favored by the light sensitive and those who cannot tolerate color distortion or whose job requires accurate color discrimination as it absorbs equally over the whole spectrum. It is not the contrast enhancer. It is a good tint for light sensitive people and for jobs which requires accurate color discrimination. A preference to grey implies light sensitivity.

Polaroid Lens

Polaroid lenses work similar to a venetian blind by only letting in light at certain angles and protecting them from the effect of glare. Without the sun's glare, objects become more distinct and are seen in their true colors. Reduced glare off water, roads, and other objects make the polarized lens a favorite for many sports. Baseball is subject to a lot of glare. Glare can make it difficult to see the ball coming at you from an inside fastball, hard-hit line drive or towering pop-up. A headache from glare can ruin your day. Golfers have to deal with the performance-killing distraction of glare from water hazards, bunkers and flat areas. Driving in glare can be risky, and road cyclists know how glare can hide potholes and other dangers. Any skier or snowboarder can tell you how glare distracts, diminishes mental focus and drains energy with tension. Fishing sessions can be futile when blinding rays bounce off water. These athletes may be highly benefitted by the use of Polaroid lenses. The additional density of silver mirror front complimented by back anti-reflection coating can be a great for sunny day events.

Photochromatic Lenses

In changeable weather conditions or in sport where you are moving from areas of bright light to shade, for example golf and cycling photochromic lenses are useful. These lenses darken in bright light and become paler in less intense light conditions.

Table 9.3 gives interesting information.

Coating

The new advanced lens coatings are very effective to improve the mechanical and optical properties of the optical lenses. Therefore, a consideration to following types is quite relevant in sports vision dispensing:

Hard Coating

Resin materials are usually softer and prone to scratches. Hard coating is a procedure to restrict scratches. A thin layer of material usually 0.5 micron to 10 micron thick is applied to the lens surface. The most common material used is lacquer which is applied either by dipping or by spinning procedure. It may be tintable or nontintable. Nontintable hard coating offers more scratch resistance than the tint able. It is not possible to see the layer of hard coating except of the edges of bifocal segments and there is no optical effect of hard

Table 9.3: Sports specific tint preference.

Sports	*Choice of lens color*	*Reason*
Golf	Brown or copper tints	These colors enhance the contrast of the ball against the green background
Cycling	Gray or green tints	Offer good color perception and reduce brightness without distorting the colors of traffic signals
Tennis	Yellow or orange tints	They can improve contrast and depth perception on the court
Water sports	Polarized sunglasses with brown, or copper tints	Reduces glare from water surfaces and enhancing visibility beneath the water's surface
Running	Gray or brown tints	They provide balanced light reduction without significant color distortion
Winter sports	Rose or pink tints	For better visibility in low-light, overcast conditions
Shooting	Yellow or orange tints	Improve contrast and target visibility, especially in low-light conditions
Basketball	Gray or brown tints	Reduces glare from indoor lights while maintaining color perception
Hiking	Green or brown tints	Hikers generally prefer for their versatility in various lighting conditions

coating if the refractive index of the lacquer used is same as that of the base lens material. If the refractive index differs, there is a change in surface reflection. The benefits of hard coating are it facilitates lens cleaning and minimizes probable scratches. There is no optical effect of hard coating if the refractive index of the lacquer used is same as that of the base lens material.

Anti-reflection Coating

Anti-reflection coating improves light transmission and thus improves the visual performance through lenses resulting in improved contrast sensitivity. It is particularly important in poor light conditions or if one eye has particular problem. In addition it also increases the cosmetic look of the lenses. When the light enters an optical medium, the speed with which it travels changes that creates surface reflection. Surface reflection results in loss of light transmission. The higher the index of the lens material, the greater is the surface reflection. Anti-reflection coating reduces reflection and thereby increases the light transmission through the lens material. However, lower surface reflection, the visible dirt and surface defects are more visible and it is more difficult to keep the lens looking clean.

Anti-static Coating

Anti-reflection coated lens surface shelters dust particles on its surface, which may result in scratches during lens cleaning. This develops the need for antistatic coating. Anti-static coating makes the surface dust repellent and facilitates clear vision by preventing accumulation of dust particles over the lens surface. This makes your glasses easier to clean as well as better to look through without any annoying dust particles in your line of vision or out of the corner of your eye.

Water-repellent Coating

A water-repellent coating literally stops water droplets from sticking to the lenses. The hydrophobic performance of the lens is achieved by having a very slight angle which effectively lets the water slide down and off. This option is perfect for those that wear their glasses at all times, as rain can often be a nuisance that obscures your vision. This problem can be eased if a hydrophobic coating is applied to the lens surface. The basic principle is to create a high surface wetting angle, which allows the water or oil to run off rather than wetting and then drying on the surface. It can be applied simply by dipping process. Baking after dipping enhances the life. It can also be applied in the vacuum chamber as the final stage of the multilayer anti-reflection coating process. The advantage it keep lens clean and protects anti-reflection coating.

Smudge-resistance Coating

A smudge-resistant coating will do just as it says. Marks such a fingerprints will not show up on the lens, allowing you to have a clear vision throughout the day. The science behind the technology is that the anti-smudge layer was developed by using perfluorinated polymers which are applied directly after the final antireflection layer using a vacuum deposition process. This may sound complicated, but what it means is unmatched clarity of vision when it comes to your glasses.

Mirror Coating

Mirror coatings on the lens not only look good but also provide a variety of visual benefits. Mirror lenses have changed considerably in recent years as technology has made it possible to create nearly limitless mirror colors and densities. Today's mirrors offer a broad range of possibilities and improved optical performance for both prescription and non-prescription wearers. Sure, colored mirror coatings are prevalent on sports lenses, and flash coatings have found a fashion home on lenses, but there are also some medical conditions that benefit from mirror coatings. The flash mirror coating creates a dynamic effect because the lenses appear to change color depending on how the light hits them. The latest trend in mirror coated lenses is the lightly visible "clear" mirror. Mirror coatings have become hugely popular on sports performance sun wear. Their color and density are matched with the base lens color's tint to enhance the wearer's visual comfort and performance. You'll find mirror tints specifically designed for water sports, land sports, snow sports, general sports, and bright sun. Light transmission in a mirror coated lens is reduced because of the high percentage of light being reflected.

An objection to absorption tinted lenses is that energy absorbed is transferred into heat which might irradiate the eyes. Using of mirror coating, the energy is reflected away from the eye thereby eliminating the possibility of irradiation by the filter itself.

Lens Material

Polycarbonate material has been the material of choice for sports vision dispensing. This is nearly ten-time impact resistant than CR 39 lenses. It has an added advantage of being very light and high refractive index. It is relatively softer material and usually comes with superior hard coating which makes it little prone to scratches. But its protective characteristics far outweighs these disadvantages. Besides, Trivex is another lens material which is nearly as tough as polycarbonate. The higher abbe value 46 improves the visual performance of the lenses through it periphery. From the point of dispensing care should be taken to ensure that the lens surface is not scratched and pitted because they affect both optical and impact resistance properties of the lenses.

■ CONTACT LENSES

Contact lenses are one of the most important modes of vision correction in sports. Usually contact lenses are the choice of correction in sports often in combination with prescription and plano appliance. The exception is the aiming sports where shooting spectacles are preferable.

In sports vision practice it is to be remembered that contact lenses are not fitted to athletes but the athletes are fitted to contact lenses. This is because some athletes will tolerate lenses better than others regardless of conditions or the sports.

The following considerations are important before fitting lenses:
- Sports and the position of athlete in the sports
- Risk of trauma which may be very common in dynamic sports, e.g., soccer or hockey
- Indoor environment with no air flow and low humidity and outdoor environment
- Relative risk of non-ionizing radiations
- Comfort issues which may be worst in non-dynamic sports when the eyes are static.

All these conditions must be considered in relation to the athlete's own physiology. In some situations, correction of choice may combination of contact lenses and spectacle on top, for example in swimming or sailing.

In general fitting contact lenses to athletes yield several advantages that are shown in **Figure 9.14**.

Peripheral Awareness

Nearly all sports demand good, if not superior peripheral awareness. Possessing a relatively large field of vision is obviously an asset in terms of sports performance for two simple reasons. Nature and evolution have made us more sensitive to movements in the peripheral area of the field of vision. Typically, lots of conflicting movements are often present in our peripheral field of vision. It implies, therefore, that in addition to seeing the peripheral area of the field of vision, an awareness of the objects in the periphery is equally important.

Since contact lenses move with the eyes, they provide an excellent macular field of vision. On the contrary, glasses are paired with the head where the lens edge and the frame also limit the field of vision. In sports like basketball and football, both offensive and defensive players must be aware of where the ball is, where their teammates are, and where the opponents are always. This suggests that a larger range of field is a factor that greatly contributes to good sporting performance in these events.

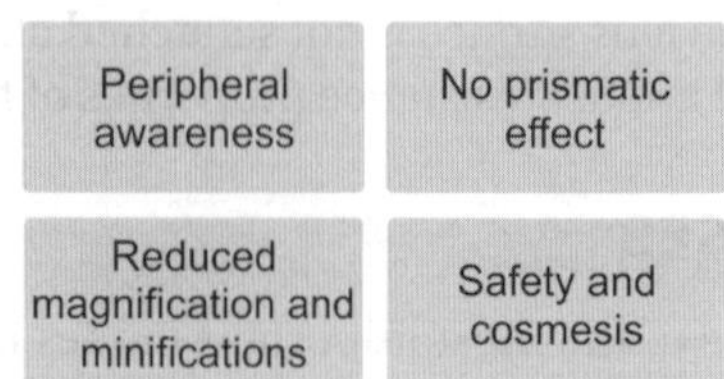

Fig. 9.14: Advantages of contact lenses.

No Prismatic Effect

Observing through an eccentric zone of the lens creates a prismatic effect, which leads to deviation similar to heterophoria that the individual tries to compensate with their own binocular fusion. This phenomenon may cause:

- Strain, if the deviation is moderate, or in other words, if the individual's capacity is good.
- Asthenopia or diplopia, if the deviation is greater. The result is observed as an increase in fixation disparity or unstable fixation disparity, which ultimately affects stereopsis adversely.

Since contact lenses do not significantly decentralize with respect to the individual's visual axis, no undesirable prismatic effects occur. This is particularly important in the case of anisometropia.

Reduced Magnifications and Minifications

A minus spectacle lens makes objects in the field of view appear smaller whereas a plus prescription makes objects look larger in the field of view. These changes are further aggravated when the refractive error is significantly higher. This is due to the vertex distance. Sometimes it may create difficulties for an individual to move about in his environment without considering a short period of adaptation. With contact lenses, however, the objects are not so much magnified or minified as they lie on pupillary plane. So, this is an important criterion to select a vision correction mode for an athlete. However, if someone who is habituated to use spectacle may find it difficult to adjust to contact lenses when fine judgment of depth is required. For instance, in table tennis the timing of a top spin smash relies critically on the distance of the bat from the ball where half of a millimeter can have drastic effect on the timing.

Safety and Cosmesis

Cosmesis is all about appearance and look. How an individual looks to him and others is important, this is natural and cannot be ignored. There is no right and wrong when it comes to cosmetics. Some people feel that they look good in spectacles, while others take spectacles as the stealer of their personality. If an athlete doesn't wear a correction modality just because he feels that he doesn't look good, it would defeat the whole purpose sports vision evaluation. This seems true also as playing sport is a social activity as much as an expression of competitive needs. The mode of correction which is cosmetically not appealing will detract the pleasure of the game. Another perception that has been seen to dominate the people's mind is that a product that looks good also performs better. It is coincidence that sports frame has part of their appeal routed in their fashion appeal. Contact lenses have the intrinsic advantage of not affecting the appearance of the athlete. When soft lenses are used for swimming, they also give a degree of protection from chemicals in the water. If lenses are disposed off after swimming, chemicals absorbed by the lenses do not remain in contact with cornea any longer. Hence it could

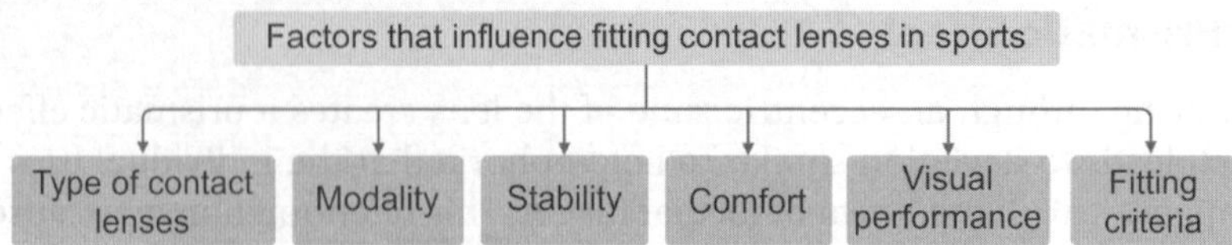

Fig. 9.15: Factors that affect contact lens fitting to athletes.

be argued that this is an advantage of wearing clean daily disposable contact lenses for swimming.

The factors as shown in **Figure 9.15** influence fitting of contact lenses in sports.

Type of Contact Lenses

Broadly there are two types of contact lenses:

1. Rigid gas permeable (RGP)
2. Soft contact lenses (SCL)

RGP lenses provide better visual acuity but the level of comfort is less as compared to SCL. There is an adaptation period of time which is quite significant and the wearer may feel the effect of glare and flare in dim light conditions. SCL improves peripheral vision and is more comfortable. Most wearers adapt to SCL very quickly. SCL are the lenses of choice in sports.

Modality

The modality of contact lenses depends upon the duration of the sports and sporting environment. For example, in water sports like swimming or sailing the first choice of modality is daily disposable lenses. Risk of *Acanthamoeba* infection and chemical keratitis is unavoidable in swimming pool. The soft contact lenses absorb the contents of the water and if it is used for long, it could adversely affect, making daily disposable the lens of choice.

Stability

The need for stability affects the lens choice and fitting criteria. SCL in fresh water (hypotonic) sticks to cornea due to passage of water into the cornea and it floats away in salt water (hypertonic). This can be used to advantage in sports like canoeing, sailing and water polo—if the lens sticks to right place. There might be situations where contact lens may not be the correction of choice.

Comfort

Contact lens discomfort is a condition characterized by episodic or persistent adverse ocular sensations related to lens wear, either with or without visual disturbance, resulting from reduced compatibility between the contact lens and the ocular environment which may include eyes stinging, burning, itching, or other eye pain abnormal feeling of something in the eye, excessive watering of the eyes. Low humidity and no air flow in indoor environment may reduce wearing comfort. Static eye may also lead to reduction in lens wearing comfort.

Visual Performance

Contact lenses can affect contrast sensitivity, but this is far outweighed by the correction that can be achieved with them especially when the refractive error is small. Contact lenses are the ideal way of dealing with small refractive errors. Small cylinders can also lead to constant searching for clarity and spasm and can often be conveniently corrected by spherical contact lenses. Contact lenses are best for monocular refractive error correction. Strong dominant athletes find significant improvement in anticipation, i.e., to judge depth. However, care should be taken while fitting contact lenses as transient instability of vision post blink is critical in sports where static visual acuity is critical. Loose fitting lenses causes more decrement.

Fitting Criteria

Stability of contact lenses on the cornea is very important for accurate and undistorted vision. So large diameter and steep fitting is advised for the duration of the game. Athlete may be informed that separate pair of contact lens needs to be used during sports which are not needed otherwise.

Contact lenses can be lost in many competitive contact sports, especially some water sports where contact lenses can be contraindicated. Sport is not always clean and clinical and hands that get muddy or faces that get muddy make contact lens wear even more problematic. It is, therefore, important to consider the environment in which the athlete plays. Cold environments are often associated with low humidity, which in turn tends to induce lens dehydration. It suggests that low water content lenses will provide maximum resistance to lens dehydration. At high altitude temperature falls and partial pressure of oxygen in the atmosphere decreases which suggests that high Dk lenses are essential for good ocular health. RGP lenses are prone to trap debris beneath the lenses and are clearly contraindicated in dirty and dusty environment. Aquatic environment is not suitable for contact lenses. Contact lenses are likely to increase the rate of infection. In fresh water chlorinated pool there is a risk of Acanthamoeba infection. Halophilic organisms pose greater threat of infection in marine water. High water content lenses are contraindicated in marine due to salt environment.

LASER TREATMENT

Tiger woods has a positive life-changing effect after having laser treatment on his eyes. Laser is also being considered as one of the modes of vision correction in sports. The debate over long-term effect of laser is still ongoing, but evidence available so far does point to long- and short-term effects which potentially do reduce visual acuity and contrast sensitivity. It is important the practitioner keeps an open mind so that the athlete can be advised in an unbiased and positive way. However, there are certain reported adverse effects of laser treatment also which must be kept in mind:

- Dry eyes
- Aberrations
- Reduced visual acuity
- Scarring
- Increased risk of trauma
- Retinal problem
- Psychological disturbances
- Glare
- Haloes
- Residual prescription
- Prescription regression
- Microtome debris
- Flap problem

Contrary to popular mythology - having the laser treatment procedure does not mean that you no longer need spectacle or contact lenses. Arguably in a sporting context, this becomes even more important than ever.

Rugby is not a game to play with either spectacle or contact lenses. Heavy weight boxers are not right candidate to wear either contact lenses or spectacles. Footballers are not allowed to wear spectacles.

It is, therefore, not wise to wipe off the scope of laser surgery from sports vision practice. It may be used effectively with fine tuning with contact lenses or spectacle.

Protection

Sports have been identified as the most common cause of severe eye injury. Safety is therefore also a primary concern in sports. The best way of avoiding ocular trauma is to avoid It., so everything that can be done to protect and enhance has a bearing on safety. This in turn would allow for a longer sporting life. Protection is another very important objective of sport vision dispensing. Eye protection depends primarily on avoidance. The main source of traumatic injury comes from direct blow to the eye or the adnexa. The use of protective appliances is one of the ways of prolonging safe and enjoyable participation in sports.

Squash

Squash balls are likely to attain the velocity up to 135 mph and may cause serious eye trauma with possibility to penetrate the orbital cavity. Both racquet and ball can cause injury. Possibility of injury increases in doubles as two players occupy the same court. These injuries can be easily prevented by the use of safety appliances.

Badminton

The shuttlecock in badminton has a diameter of 0.75 inches and can easily penetrate the orbital opening. Wearing approved safety appliances can prevent these possible injuries easily.

Boxing

Boxing is clearly played with an intension to injure. Damage to eyes in boxing can result from direct blow or from shock waves. Depending upon the force of the blow damage may result in injury to retina, eyelids etc.

Rugby

Physical clashes with opponent's hands, elbows, feet or sometimes fists can hit the eyes accidentally and cause injuries. Deliberate hit with hands are quite common in rugby. That is why widespread use of helmet in very common in rugby.

Basketball

Eye injuries are quite common in basketball due to fingers and elbows rather than ball. Common injuries include eyelid abrasion or laceration, orbital contusions and fractures and corneal abrasions.

Golf

Golf-related ocular injuries are rare. However, both golf ball and the golf club head are quite hard and can directly transmit a large amount of force to the globe.

Ice Hockey

In ice hockey, the most common cause of injury is from the stick coming in between face and face protector. Puck may also cause eye injury.

Swimming

Swimming do not present a significant risk of eye injury. Swimming goggles can potentially cause a blunt trauma injury if they slip during removal or when put on. The elastic band can cause the goggles to snap back and cause severe injuries.

Cosmetics

Good looks are a snare that everyone desires to be caught in, and athletes are no exception to this general rule. Therefore, it is up to the optometrist to ensure that the interests of the athletes are optimized. If an appliance caters to the aesthetic aspirations of the athlete, they are more likely to use it, ultimately leading to the achievement of objectives. Otherwise, the athlete may avoid using the appliance altogether.

In sports vision practice, it is crucial not to limit oneself to one mode of correction. Before any decision is made about the option, the nature of the sport itself has to be carefully considered. Correction also depends on whether the sport involves aiming or anticipating movements. The ophthalmological significance of eye injuries is self-evident. Optometrically, it could be argued that good vision and peripheral awareness help to avoid such injuries. For instance, seeing the cricket ball early provides extra time to take evasive action, while noticing the movement of a squash racket in peripheral vision might help to prevent serious injuries. In sports vision, safety is paramount. Sport vision makes no compromises when it comes to ensuring the safety of athletes.

Visual Demands in Tennis

10 CHAPTER

TERMINOLOGIES

Ace, Serve, Stance, Rally, Topspin, Net, Deuce, Double Fault, Crosscourt, Backhand, Forehand, Baseline, etc.

Tennis is a dynamic sport and is played with a racket and a ball on a court divided by a net. It can be played by two players or four players. When it is played by two players, it is called singles match and when it is played by four players, it is called doubles match. Players take the position on both the sides of the net use a racquet to hit the ball back and forth to each other. The object is to propel the ball over the net in such a way that it bounces in court and beats any attempt by an opponent to return it.

Tennis is played by both men and women on varieties of court surfaces. The size of the court varies depending on whether a singles or doubles match is being played, but the height of the net is constant. Each player has a stringed racket especially designed for tennis to hit a hollow rubber ball. Play begins with a service, each player serving in turn for one game. The opponent returns the ball across the net so that it falls within the other player's court. The ball is allowed to bounce only once after being struck. The player scores a point when the ball bounces twice in court or lands outside the court or misses the ball or causes the ball to hit the net or when a rally is broken.

Tennis is predominantly an anticipatory sport (**Fig. 10.1**). In tennis the ball has to travel only 24 meters before it reaches the returning player. The

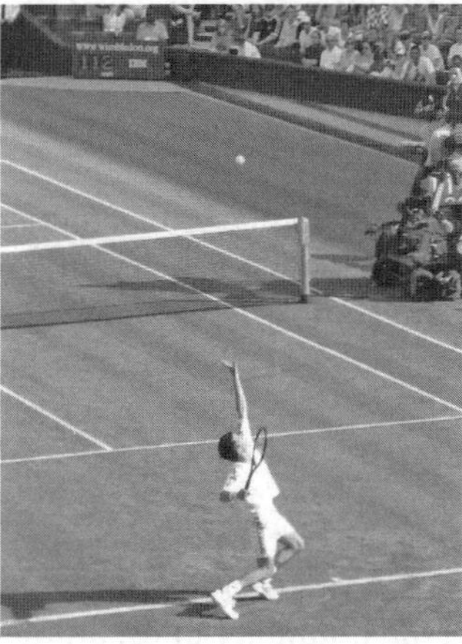

Fig. 10.1: Anticipating to aim the racket to serve.

speed of ball traveling makes anticipation very important visual element. In fact, the evidence suggests that for a ball served at 150 kms per hour, the responding player only gets half a second to determine the speed, direction and spin of the ball before executing the shot. Accurate anticipation relies on two forms of information—prior information, based on knowledge of how a particular opponent usually plays and detection of visual cues that predict the direction and force of the opponent's response. Angle of the racket head is the principal visual cue used in tennis. The ability to anticipate what is about to happen and when, provides a distinct edge to a player over another. Together with anticipation, there is a residual aiming requirement when the racket is directly in line with the aiming eye as it might be during a serve or a hit. While aiming, generally there is an alignment. When a team player hits, alignment is missing, but in serve and volley arm and the ball are relatively in alignment, nearly halfway status between true aiming and no aiming at all. In tennis, the player constantly focuses on the net with fixing bars at the two sides. This gives the cues to the position in relation to opponent and the aim is achieved with body alignment with the net. Hence aiming is not very important and is achieved using the subliminal cues. The importance of various elements of visual system in Tennis can be understood by following description:

VISUAL ACUITY

Tennis is a fast-moving sport where either the target is in motion or the player is in motion and the time available to the player to react is very short, requiring fast reaction time. Dynamic Visual acuity is very important and since it is played with color ball and a specific background, there is a good demand for contrast between the two. Static visual acuity is critical while fixation during serve. Small target size, speed of the target and the player and a great demand for anticipation introduce some very complex visual equation for the brain to compute. If vision is degraded, it may disrupt aiming and thereby performance. Color vision is not very critical as it is played with predetermined set of colors.

ACCOMMODATION–VERGENCE FUNCTION

The player who is serving needs to focus on immediate target and then to opponent's position at the opposite end to place his shot. The receiver, on the other hand, has to focus on the server's racket, his body movement and then to fast approaching ball. The player has to have the ability to shift the focus rapidly throughout the contest even during general body stamina is running down due to heavy exertion. Poor focusing ability will severely affect anticipation and poor convergence will affect aiming.

OCULOMOTOR SKILL

Fixation is critical in serving the ball. Quick, accurate saccades are needed to follow the rapidly changing location of the player and movement of the ball in relation to the net and the boundary lines. Studies have shown that if the head has to move to aid ball tracking, it will not only reduce stamina, but will also affect the balance.

DEPTH PERCEPTION

Tennis is predominantly anticipatory sport; hence good depth perception is by far the biggest visual attribute of the elite tennis player. Anticipating the speed and the direction of the ball and also to judge whether the ball will land in or out of the court boundaries are important visual skills **(Fig. 10.2)**. This is also critical for accurate shot placements and becomes most important during serve to keep the spatial awareness of the tossed ball so that the racket is correctly aimed at the ball in right time.

BINOCULAR VISION

A perfectly balanced binocular vision is very critical visual skill in tennis as it affects depth perception which has a direct bearing on anticipation. Since tennis is predominantly anticipatory sport, binocular vision will immediately affect the performance. This is also important visual skill to have the awareness of complete playing court and the position of the opponent so that the return shot can be placed to the advantage. Importance of contrast also necessitates good binocular vision.

CENTRAL-PERIPHERAL AWARENESS

The player must concentrate centrally on the opponent's court position and the possible direction of the ball which will come off his opponent's racket. Meanwhile he must be peripherally aware of where the net and the boundary lines of the court are. It helps in picking up lob shots when running backwards while looking over your shoulder. However, in doubles the player must have additional peripheral awareness of his partner's body and racket to avoid collision and injury.

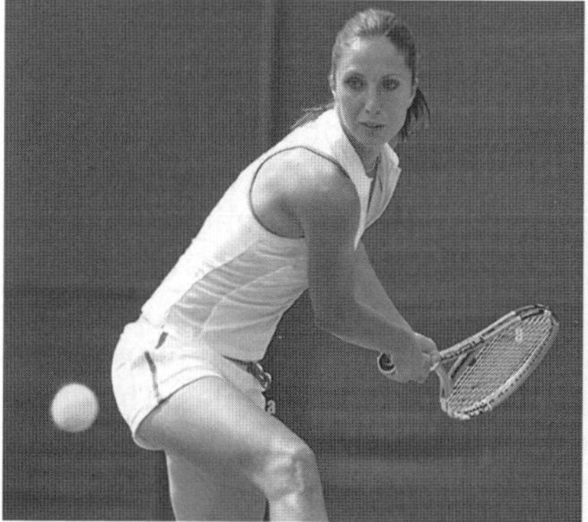
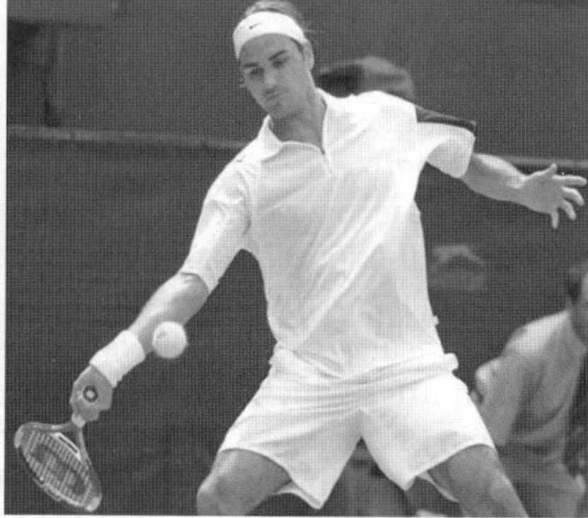

Fig. 10.2: Depth perception—anticipating the speed and the direction of the ball.

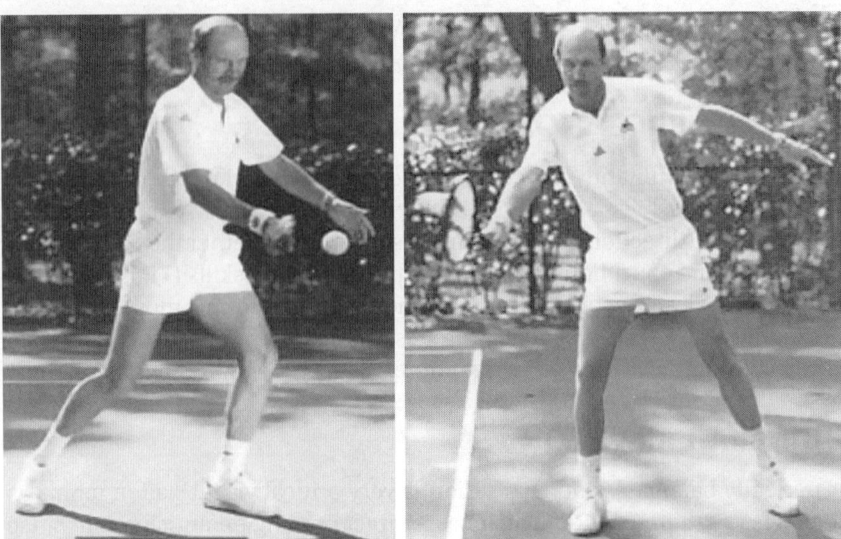

Fig. 10.3: Fast detection of approaching ball to bring hand in line with its direction.

EYE-HAND COORDINATION

In tennis the eyes detect the position of the fast-approaching ball, the information of which is transported via optic nerve towards the central nervous system. The incoming information is identified by comparison with past experiences, allowing for a decision on the most appropriate response. Once the movement sequence or motor program has been selected, the motor neurons transport the relevant information to the muscular system, where information about the force and timing of muscular movements allows for an efficient response **(Fig. 10.3)**. All the above procedure happens very quickly; the novice or average player takes time to organize his response. He may seem fast, but not quick enough to beat an elite competitor. The speed of tennis necessitates fast eye-hand coordination.

GLARE RECOVERY

Mostly tennis is played outdoors under bright sunlight condition. So, lob shots may get lost in the sun momentarily, if dazzle is caused to the retina. The player must recover quickly before the next return shot is imminent. Longer duration of the sport also necessitates glare protection as it causes headaches, visual fatigue and impairs vision.

The optical dispensing in tennis is also important because of probable ocular injuries which can occur at the net specially in doubles. They may also occur because of a miss-hit or partner's racket. Therefore, use of contact lenses is more appropriate than spectacles for vision correction.

Visual Demands in Table Tennis

11 CHAPTER

TERMINOLOGIES

Racket, Serve, Paddle, Stroke, Spin, Smash, Loop, Lob, Game point, Forehand, Backhand, Chop, Block

Table Tennis is a fast-paced indoor sport that requires individual skill and excellent eye-hand coordination. The key skills for a successful Table Tennis player includes racket bounce, forehand volley, backhand volley and serving. It is a non-weather dependent sport having specific requirements regarding size of hall, lighting, flooring, etc., depending upon the level of the competition. The ball used in Table Tennis is a light object and its flight can be easily affected by the gusts of air or the spin of the ball **(Fig. 11.1)**.

Table Tennis is a visually demanding sport. Speed and direction of racket is the principal visual cue used in Table Tennis. Watching the ball and the bat is the best way to make sure that the bat goes to exactly where the ball is. Watch the ball closely from the time the opponent hits the ball until it hits your own bat. It is also important to be watching the opponent and what he is doing, in order to plan where you are going to hit the ball. Otherwise, you are likely to hit a great shot right to where the opponent is waiting for it. Watching the opponent and anticipating his defensive position are equally important to have an idea of what shot he is going to play next. Thus, anticipation is more predominant in table tennis. Every time the player anticipates the speed, spin and the direction of the shot to aim his bat to execute the return shot. Opponents position, net and the size of the table facilitate aiming during return shot. Aiming is also needed while serving to bring the bat to the line of the ball and place the serve to your advantage. The importance of various elements of visual system in table tennis can be understood by following description:

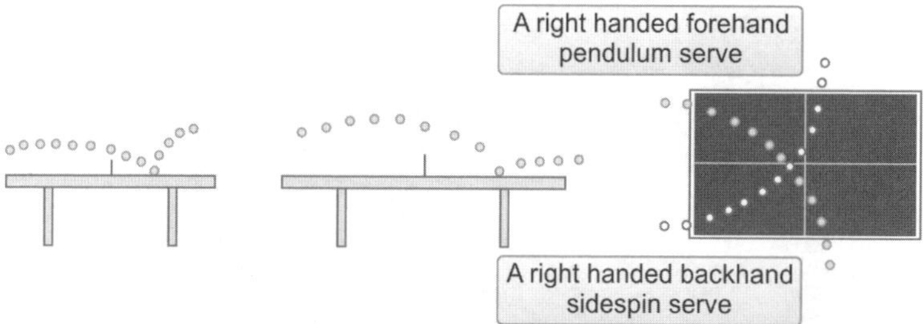

Fig. 11.1: Different types of serves and shots in Table Tennis.

VISUAL ACUITY

Once you hit the ball, you need to watch the opponent closely up until he makes contact with the ball. Then you should be watching the ball closely up until you hit it again, and once you have hit again, you should go back to watching the opponent again, until he makes contact with the ball and so on **(Fig. 11.2)**. Every time the player needs to watch either the fast-moving ball or the opponent in motion or he himself is moving. So Dynamic Visual Acuity is very critical in Table Tennis, as either the target is moving or the observer is in motion. A Table Tennis player tracks the objects with different speed and at different distances. Table Tennis is played indoors in low illumination. In low illumination there is a tendency for the Purkinje shift, i.e., the peak sensitivity of the human eye shifts towards the blue end of the color spectrum, thereby reducing the contrast. An expert Table Tennis player will definitely develop better acuity in reduced illumination than a non-player. The importance of contrast becomes more critical to have a good discrimination between ball color and the table color. Color vision is not terribly critical as the ball is easily contrasted against table. The small target size, high target speed and the need for good contrast establishes the huge demand on good visual acuity in table tennis. Research has shown that visual acuity in reduced illumination in Table Tennis players has been found to be developed significantly.

ACCOMMODATION–VERGENCE FUNCTION

Table Tennis player should fixate on a small ball that moves very rapidly in free space with lack of spatial clues from opponent's court to your court. Additionally, he should see the opponent and the table simultaneously. Saccadic eye movement fixates only at the first and the last point of fixation. Therefore, accommodative system should follow fixation point appropriately.

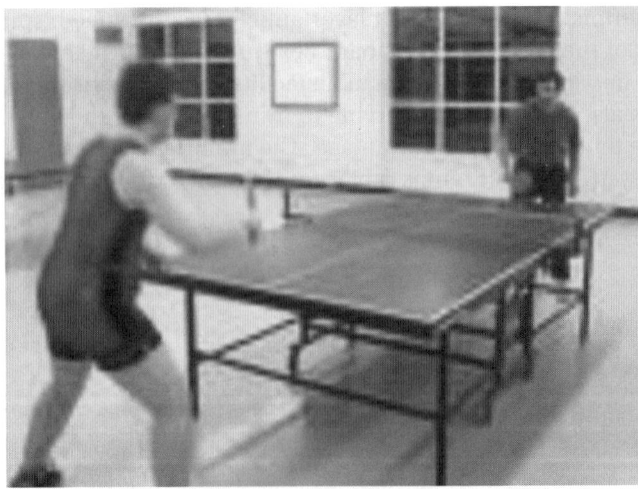

Fig. 11.2: Watching the ball and opponent's movement.

As the ball approaches towards you, the eye quickly focuses and converges. After striking the ball, the eyes diverge and relax accommodation very rapidly to follow the flight of the ball and the positions of the opponent. So, there is a huge role of accommodative convergence and divergence. The player has to be able to shift focus from near to far or intermediate targets rapidly throughout the contest, while the general body stamina is running down due to heavy exertion.

OCULOMOTOR SKILL

The ocular motor skill is highly critical in Table Tennis to track the high speed spinning ball properly and to communicate its relative position in the space to the neuromuscular system to position the bat to make contact. In Table Tennis, the fixation points changes as fast as the ball and the position of the opponent. The velocity of the ball is very high and the eyes should see it clearly. Therefore, any player who can follow the ball as fast as possible, he would be more successful. Saccadic eye movement are used for fixation on the ball. Suppression takes place in saccadic eye movements. Only the first and the last point of fixation can be seen, and the saccadic pathway is suppressed. Therefore, the first and the last point is very important from visual acuity point of view **(Fig. 11.3)**. Smooth pursuit movement is not that important.

DEPTH PERCEPTION

In Table Tennis the player should anticipate the speed of the ball, its spin and the direction of opponent's stroke and the spatial judgement of the ball in a short time. The player also needs to know the correct spot to place his shot

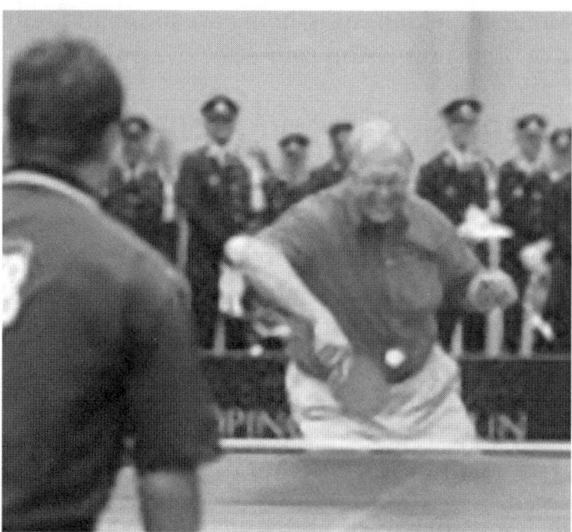

Fig. 11.3: Saccadic eye movement for fixation.

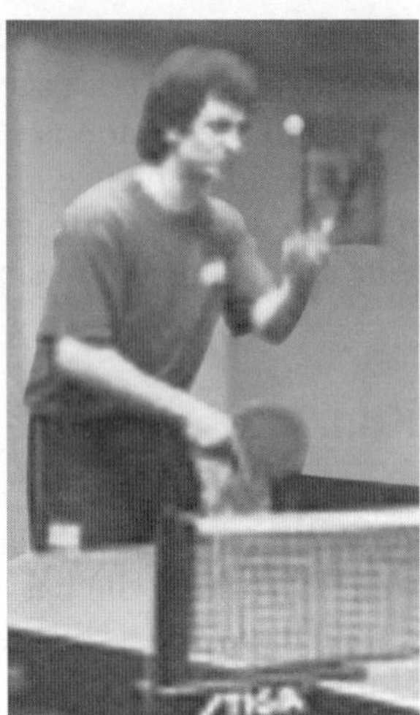

Fig. 11.4: Spatial judgement of ball.

and to judge whether to play the shot with back-hand or forehand or leave it. Thus, he uses depth perception to decide how to play a shot most effectively. Depth perception is also important when the ball is tossed high up in the air before serving **(Fig. 11.4)**.

BINOCULAR VISION

The huge demand of focus flexibility, high contrast, good visual acuity with the need of some peripheral awareness, make binocular vision an important visual need for Table Tennis player. Any anomaly in binocular vision will disrupt body balance and cause anomalies of accommodation which in turn will affect performance. Table Tennis, being predominantly anticipatory sport, the importance of binocular vision cannot be overruled.

CENTRAL-PERIPHERAL AWARENESS

The Table Tennis player should also be using his peripheral vision when hitting the ball to get an idea of where the opponent is moving to and where he may be vulnerable. Central-peripheral vision should be much better at locating a faraway slow-moving opponent in relation to a static table and then tracking a close up fast moving ball in relation to yourself. This skill is especially critical in doubles when already fairly small playing area becomes more congested to avoid collision and injury.

EYE-HAND CO-ORDINATION

An expert Table Tennis player should anticipate ball trajectory, direction of opponent's stroke and opponent's stroke movement and accordingly aim his own bat at the ball to execute his counter stroke. During all such processes

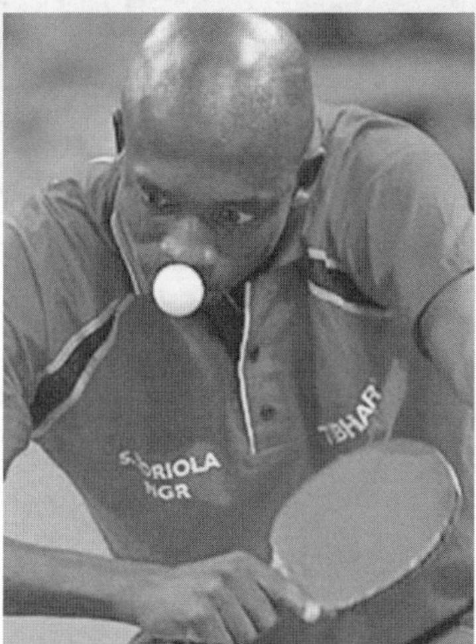

Fig. 11.5: Anticipating ball trajectory to execute his shot.

the velocity of the ball is very high and the eye should see it clearly, so that the player can hit the ball successfully. So eye-hand coordination is not only very important in Table Tennis but it has to be very fast. The Table Tennis player fixates on the center of the target, i.e., ball and moves their head and eyes to search for the line before initiating motor movement of the arm or hands to hit the target **(Fig. 11.5)**. Sometimes the player may not be quick with his hand and wrist, they may be fast on their feet and have excellent body balance. In table tennis balancing the body in correct position before executing the shot effectively is very critical, making eye-hand-body coordination a very important skill.

GLARE RECOVERY

Glare recovery is not too big point of concern for Table Tennis player as it is an indoor game and is played under light focused on the table right from the top of the table. General hall lights are not very bright to cause any glare. Perhaps a photophobic player may suffer glare from the lights directly or from the reflection caused by the table surface.

In Table Tennis the average total time to react to a shot is usually around 0.25 of a second. With lots of training and practice it can be reduced to 0.18 of a second. This is one of the biggest factors in what separates the greats from top players, this proves the importance of vision and visual reaction in table tennis. You need to improve your vision and visual reaction time or the speed with which your brain interprets and reacts to your opponent's action. Contact lenses are more advantageous but the choice of contact lens must be done carefully considering the effects of indoor environment.

Visual Demands in Badminton

12 CHAPTER

TERMINOLOGIES

Alley, Forehand, Hairpin net shot, Half-court shot, Net shot, Push shot, Rally, Shuttlecock, Smash, Wood shot

Badminton is a dynamic fast paced racket and shuttlecock sport played as an indoor or outdoor sport. It is played at many levels throughout the world by males or females or both together. It can be a fun game on lawn or beach or highly competitive athletic game, played at national and international levels. The object of the game is to hit the shuttlecock over the nets so that it lands in the opponent's court before it can be returned. The important shots to achieve the object are serve, forehand, backhand, smash, delicate touch and so on. The rally begins with a serve and is broken when the shuttlecock falls on the court or outside the court or at the nets and thus the point is scored.

Badminton is predominantly an anticipatory sport **(Fig. 12.1)**. The shuttlecock has to travel 44 feet long distance before it reaches the returnee. This makes anticipation a very important visual need. The responding player needs to anticipate the speed of the shuttlecock, its spatial location in the air and direction in a very short span of time before aiming the racket in line with the shuttlecock to hit. Like tennis, aiming is achieved with subliminal cues

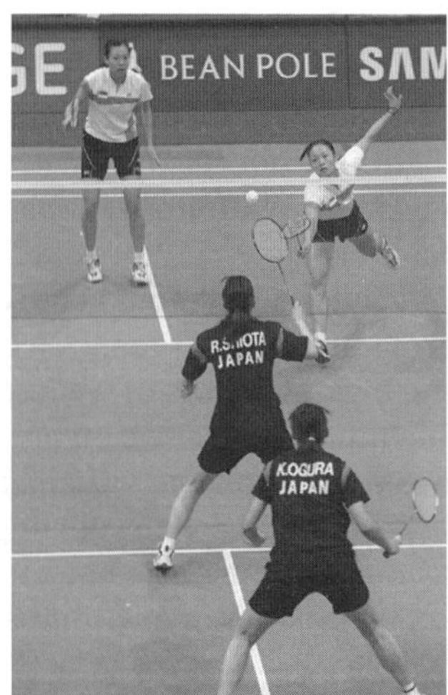

Fig. 12.1: Anticipating the shuttlecock to hit.

to the position of the opponent, net and the court side boundaries. Athlete's gaze direction is mostly used as visual cue in Badminton. Eye movement may signal the opponent's intention or it may be a bluff. Hence aiming is not very important in Badminton.

The importance of various elements of visual system in Badminton can be understood by following description:

VISUAL ACUITY

Badminton is a fast dynamic sport where either the player is in motion or the target is in motion and the time available to the player to react is very short, requiring fast reaction time **(Fig. 12.2)**. Dynamic visual acuity is more important than static visual acuity. Since it is usually played with white shuttlecock, there is a good demand for high contrast between the target and its background. Small target size, speed of the target and the need of high contrast increases the importance of good visual acuity in badminton. If the vision is interrupted because of the need for correction, it may affect anticipation and also aiming which is needed to place the shot.

ACCOMMODATION–VERGENCE FUNCTION

Rapid shift of focus at distance, near and intermediate throughout the game is critical. Moreover, long sustained focusing ability is essential because of long duration of the game. Ill-sustained focusing ability will affect athlete's performance at the later stage of the game and poor vergence will affect aiming considerably.

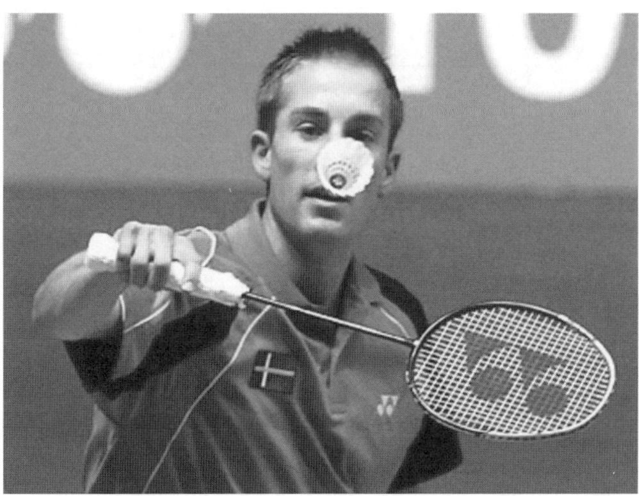

Fig. 12.2: Watching the shuttlecock in the air.

OCULOMOTOR SKILL

The speed of badminton makes oculomotor skill, a very important skill in badminton. Good, quick and accurate eye tracking ability is needed to develop the athlete's performance in badminton. Fixation is needed while serving to place it at the aimed spot. Saccades are very important to follow the fast traveling shuttle. Delicate touch placements of shots are great skill in badminton where pursuit eye movements and reflexive vestibular movements are essential.

DEPTH PERCEPTION

Badminton is predominantly an anticipatory sport in which depth perception is extremely important for accurate placement of shots, and to judge the distance and the speed of the shuttlecock **(Fig. 12.3)**. Also depth perception is needed for placing the shuttlecock at the sweet spot of the racket while hitting to have maximum power. Good depth perception is equally important to judge whether the shot is in or out the court during the rally.

BINOCULAR VISION

A good teaming of both eyes is essential in badminton to have good anticipation of the fast approaching shuttlecock. The awareness of the width of the court and opponent's position in the court are all influenced by binocular vision. The big demand of contrast in badminton because of its target color and high speed also necessitates good binocular vision.

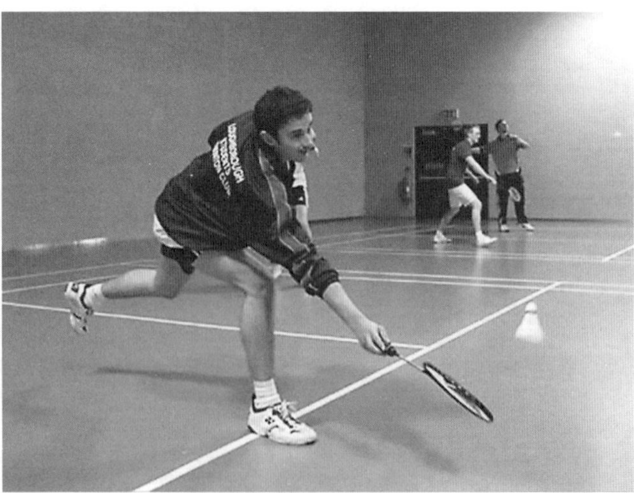

Fig. 12.3: Judging the speed and direction of the shuttlecock.

CENTRAL-PERIPHERAL AWARENESS

The player must fixate centrally on the opponent's court position and on his racket and torso and at the same time he must be peripherally aware of the net and the boundary lines of the court to place his shot correctly. Peripheral awareness in badminton is more important especially in high tossed returns. Besides, awareness of partner's body and his racket in doubles is also needed.

EYE-HAND-BODY COORDINATION

Badminton is characterized by fast movement from front to back and from one side to another while looking at the shuttlecock in the air **(Fig. 12.4)**. In fact, there is a good demand for eye and entire body coordination as the shots are executed once the body is positioned correctly. The faster the eye communicates the signals to the central nervous system to bring the body into position, the more reaction time is available to the player to execute the shot.

GLARE RECOVERY

Now-a-days elite class badminton is mostly played indoors in artificial diffuse lights, therefore, glare is not a big issue. However, if it is played outside in the sun, the players must be able to recover fast from dazzling sun while negotiating with a high tossed return.

The shuttlecock is one of the fastest moving racket propelled objects in sports, making it a highly visually demanding sport. It requires fast eyes and also fast head movements while keeping the clear image. Although it relatively safer sport. But the sheer speed of shuttlecock indicates the need of eye protection in badminton.

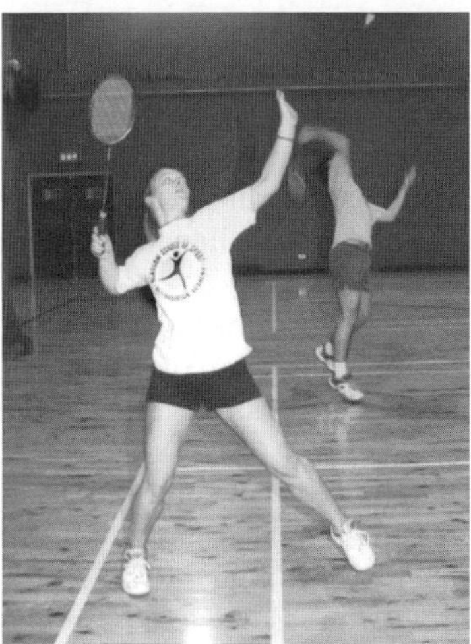

Fig. 12.4: Excellent eye-hand-body coordination.

Visual Demands in Cricket

13 CHAPTER

TERMINOLOGIES

Appeal, Boundary, Bails, Edge, Sweep, Hook shot, Yorker, Square cut, Slip, Bowler, Fielder, Batsman, Cover drive, Straight drive, Stumps, Spin, Catch

Cricket is an outdoor dynamic sport played between two teams consisting of 11 players each. The main playing arena is known as *Pitch* which is 22 yards long ,10 feet wide strip. On two ends of the pitch, a set of three stumps are dug. The two captains of teams decide their turn to bat by tossing a coin. Two umpires are stationed in the ground. The two batsman are on the pitch from the team which is batting and all eleven players are spread on the field from the team which is fielding. The match is won or lost by the runs scored by the two teams. One of the players from the fielding side bowls to the batsman who hits the ball with his bat and the rest of 10 players from fielding side fields the ball. The game basically has three different activities.

- Batting
- Bowling
- Fielding

BATTING

Probably batting is the toughest activity of the game as a small mistake can send the batsman back to the pavilion. One mistake and his life in the inning is finished. The bowler can commit mistake and the maximum penalty that he can incur is to concede a four or a six runs at the most. The batsman, therefore, must take care of the following points when the bowler runs to deliver the ball **(Fig. 13.1)**:

- Watch the ball right from the time the bowler starts to run.
- Anticipate the speed and the direction of the ball.
- Co-ordinate eye, hand and feet to strike the ball with the bat at the correct time.
- Aim the bat to bring it in line with the ball and decide the stroke.

Anticipation is the predominant visual skill in batting. The batsman looks at the bowler's torso while he is running into bowl and moves his gaze to the bowler's hand just before the ball is delivered. He needs to perceive several visual cues like bowler's action, the speed with which he swings his arm, whether he turns his body or drops his shoulder. All this information is used to

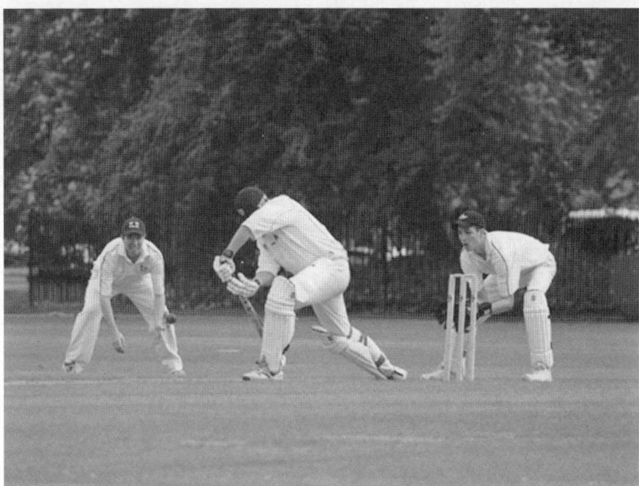

Fig. 13.1: Watch the ball, anticipating the speed, co-ordinating eye, hand and feet to aim the bat to execute the shot.

anticipate the speed, line and length of the ball. At times perfect anticipation decides the fate of a batsman in an inning. The batsman, then, brings his bat in line with the ball to hit it to complete the process of aiming. Aiming is achieved with the bowler's torso and the bowler's hand movement.

BOWLING

Bowling has basically two variables: Pace or Fast Bowling and Spin Bowling. There are innumerable variations derived from these two basic variables. The pace bowling is usually characterized by its speed which may vary between 80 to 150 kms per hour. The spin bowler runs from a shorter distance to deliver a flighted turning delivery which swings in the air as well as turns off the pitch. The bowler in fact tries to disguise his bowling action by movement pattern. The bowler needs to look at the batsman and his position constantly to aim the ball at the correct spot **(Fig. 13.2)**. Length and direction of the ball is changed by the bowler according to the weakness or strength of the batsman and also in conformity with the field. Therefore, the bowler needs to aim at merry spot that makes it predominantly an aiming activity. Aiming is achieved by the batsman stance and by anticipating the type of shot with the peripheral awareness of the field placements.

FIELDING

All the players of the fielding side are spread on the field to chase the ball hit by the batsman or to catch it in the air or to pick up and throw at the stumps **(Fig. 13.3)**. However, there are some specialized positions in the field for which the technique to field the ball is quite special. Slip fielders on the off-side should watch the ball coming down the wicket onto the bat with their

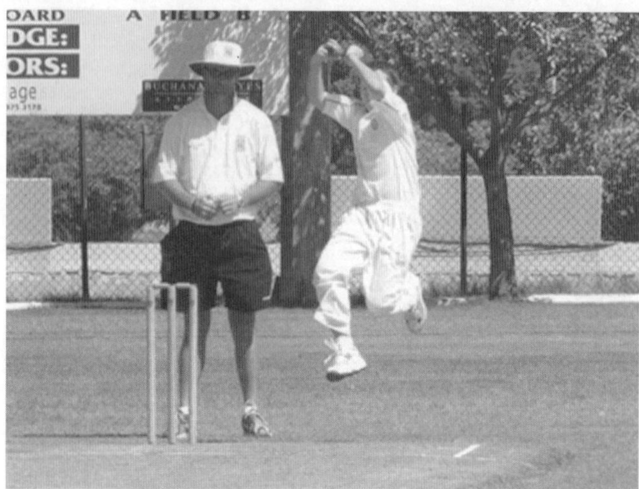

Fig. 13.2: Aiming to bowl.

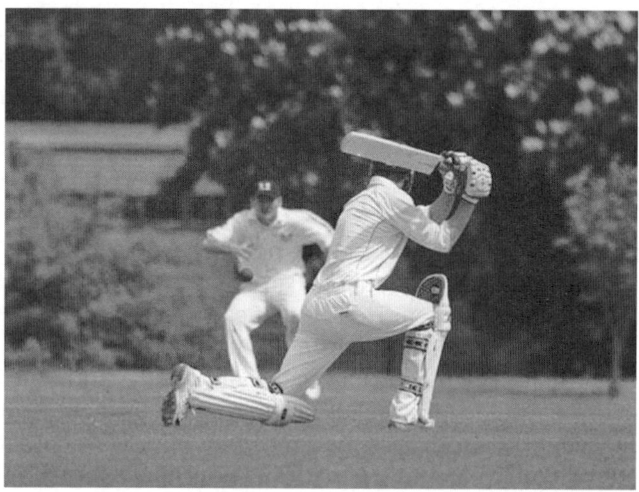

Fig. 13.3: The fielder is anticipating the direction of the shot to field the ball.

hands totally open. Close-in fielders must switch their eyes to the batsman just before the bowler releases the ball. Fielders away from the wicket must start moving in when the bowler is nearing the end of his run. The wicket keeping is very specialized position in the fielding. He must always be vigilant to get a good sight of the ball so that he can gather it quite neatly. Whatever be the position of the player in the field, anticipation seems to be predominant visual skill of the fielder at all positions. To catch the ball, the distance and speed of approach of the ball has to be judged to aim the cupped hands by lining up with the ball.

The importance of various elements of visual system in Cricket can be understood by following description:

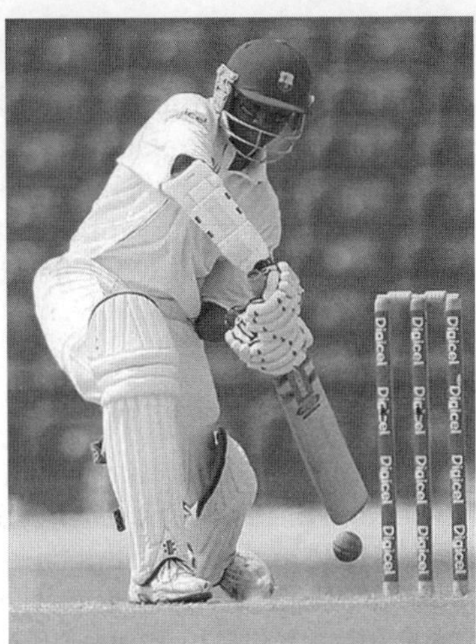

Fig. 13.4: Anticipating the speed of the approaching ball and aiming his bat to hit it.

VISUAL ACUITY

The batsman while batting looks at the running bowler, anticipate the speed of the approaching ball and aims his bat held in the hands at the ball to hit it **(Fig. 13.4)**. Dynamic visual acuity is critical because every time he is watching the object in motion-either the running bowler or the approaching ball or the hit ball or the fielder running towards the ball. Whereas the bowler runs the predetermined number of steps to throw the ball at a fixed static target, he also needs to have good dynamic visual acuity to aim the ball correctly. In fact, they need to have good distance vision so much so that they can see head pin on the pitch to aim the ball. The fielders are repeatedly looking at the batsman from their position and switch their eyes to the ball as soon as it is hit by the batsman. They need to have both good static and dynamic visual acuity. The need of high contrast also increases as the day passes. Contrast is affected by mist or fog and the game is stopped when the light level reduces below stipulated level. Color vision is not very critical.

ACCOMMODATION–VERGENCE FUNCTION

The batsman looks at the bowler's torso while he is running to deliver the bowl and will move his gaze to the bowler's hand just before the ball is delivered. Bowlers are bowling from a distance of 22 yards before which they run in from further away. Besides the batsman has to take the decision when the ball is still to travel approximately 10 meters. Decision taken later than that may not be very effective. The understanding is that the role of accommodation is almost negligible. Accommodation does not seem to have any role while bowling also. However, poor accommodative flexibility may result in poor catching while fielding.

OCULOMOTOR SKILL

Cricket is not as fast as table tennis, although the batsman needs to deal with the fast swinging ball properly from relatively static position, just by his footwork. Throughout the pathway of the ball, he needs to keep his eyes on it. So pursuit movement coupled with saccade is important in batting. Saccadic eye movement is relatively more important while fielding. But fixation ability at the target is more important for the bowlers.

DEPTH PERCEPTION

Anticipation is a primary visual skill for the batsman who anticipates the speed and direction of the ball to hit. The batsman need to develop the spatial judgement of the ball so that he can time his shot correctly. Poor timing may be associated with reduced depth perception. In cricket we often see that the batsman is deceived by the slower ball. The bowler that have success with this ball are the ones that manage to keep their action exactly as if they were going to bowl a faster ball. The batsman, anticipates a faster ball, would then make his decision as to shot that he is going to play at the moment the ball leaves the bowler's hand. By the time he realizes that it is a slower bowl, he often does not have enough time to change his decision. The consequence is that he is too early on the shot, resulting in the ball being scooped up in the air. Depth perception is very important to know the spatial location of the ball and judge its relative position and direction of it fall in the air while catching **(Fig. 13.5)**. Depth perception is not so critical while bowling which is predominantly an aiming activity.

BINOCULAR VISION

Good binocular vision is very important in cricket batting as the batsman needs to be aware of both side's field placements to execute his shot into

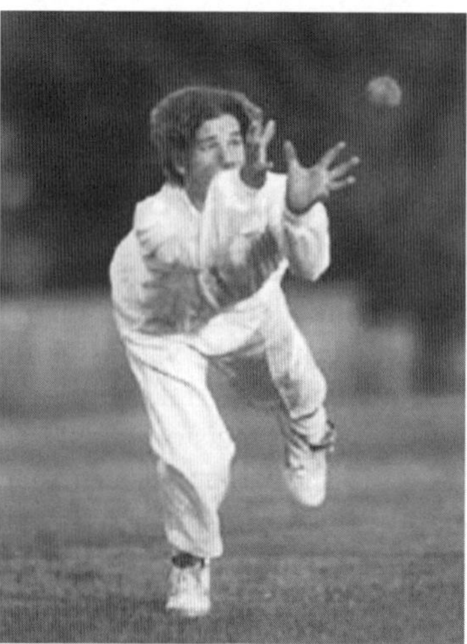

Fig. 13.5: Spatial judgement of the ball.

the gap. Two eyes must work as a pair in batting and that the dominant eye should not be hindered by facial features or head tilt. Most elite batman in the world are totally strong right dominant and favored a full on stance and straight head. Bowling, predominantly an aiming activity is favored by cross dominancy with dominant eye peeping over leading arm as in case of left eye, right hand. Unless binocular vision is established early in the life, stereopsis cannot develop which affects catching ability while fielding. Good binocular vision also enhances contrast and thereby visual acuity.

CENTRAL-PERIPHERAL AWARENESS

The batsman fixates at the bowler to face the delivery and also looks at the positions of the fielders so that he can hit at the empty area. Central-peripheral awareness is critical to achieve the result. Good peripheral vision is very important for the fielders. Central visual acuity is more important while bowling.

EYE-HAND COORDINATION

The batsman hits the ball with the bat held in the hands. He fixates on the center of the target, i.e., ball and moves his hand and eyes to search for the position before initiating motor movement of the arm or hand to hit the ball. So eye-hand coordination is not only very important in batting but it has to be very fast. Eye-hand coordination is not as important while bowling because the motor movement of the hands is initiated as soon as the number of predetermined steps is over and the bowler is onto the crease to deliver the ball. But again while fielding eyes, hand, body and foot coordination becomes very important because if the fielder cannot balance himself while running towards the ball to pick it up, he will not be able to aim at the stumps correctly.

GLARE RECOVERY

Usually cricketer use visors while batting and fielding which prevents the effect of any glare on the eyes. At times during fielding they use glare protection glasses. Fast glare recovery is very essential while catching a scooped shot. Glare recovery is not very critical issue while bowling.

In cricket batting response time needs to be related to the speed of the ball and the length of the pitch. The fast bowler delivers the ball at a speed of 80 to 150 kms per hour, implies that the response time has to be very fast—a critical factor specially while trying a hook shot. Fast response while picking up the ball and throwing at the stumps may prevent an extra run scored or may fetch a wicket to the fielding side. Fast reflexes and reactions are the traits of the great wicket keeper. Visual reaction time is not so critical for a bowler. As far as ocular injuries are concerned, ocular injuries have not been reported significantly.

Visual Demands in Baseball

14 CHAPTER

TERMINOLOGIES

Base, Bunt, Battery, Count, Diamond, Double play, Error, Fly ball, Four ball, Pinch hitter, Pinch runner, Power hitter, Relay, etc.

Baseball is one of the well-known sports within the family of bat and ball games. It is a power hitting, explosive and dynamic sport in which two teams of nine players each plays against each other. One team has possession of the ball and delivers it to one of the members of the batting team who tries to hit it. The two teams take their turn in two distinct roles one after another. The batting team tries to score runs by hitting ball with a bat which is made of narrow and round wood, while the members of the other team field the ball in an attempt to prevent scoring and put batting players out. A game of baseball consists of nine innings. The game is played on a diamond shape field, the four corners of which are home plate, first base, second base and third base **(Fig. 14.1)**. These bases are square white bags that are secured to the ground. The distance between bases is 60 feet in most soft ball league. The batter stands next to the home plate as he tries to hit the baseball. His intention is to advance around the other bases and return “home”, thus scoring a run. At around the middle of the diamond, there is a pitcher plate, which is made of rubber. The

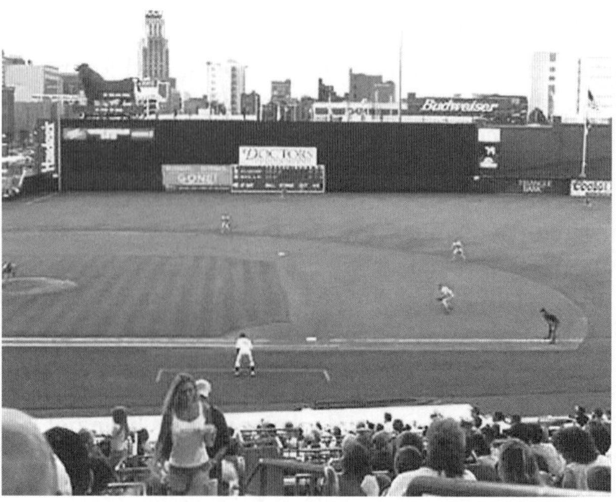

Fig. 14.1: Baseball.

pitcher has to have his one foot touching the rubber when he delivers the ball to the batter. There are basically three aspects of baseball game:

1. Batting
2. Pitching
3. Fielding

BATTING

Unlike cricket, batting in baseball is mainly characterized by power hitting. Some batters who are particularly skilled have the ability to place the hit and direct the ball to desired location. The batter **(Fig. 14.2)** needs to choose a comfortable stance among closed stance, open stance and even stance. The body weight is on rear foot with hips and shoulders are at level. Hands away from the body about 8 to 12 inches on the same plane. No matter what stance the batter is in, the trick to good hitting is getting the body right behind the line of the pitch. The ideal hitter would probably have a combination of strength, determination, coordination, confidence, vision, rhythm, style, body control, quick hands, and the will to learn and to take advice. In order to get the bat started, he moves his hands back slightly as the pitcher is getting ready to release the ball. If he likes the pitch, he goes ahead and hits it. If he doesn't like the pitch, then he holds up his swing. To accomplish this successfully the batter always keeps the eyes on the pitcher's arm and the ball, anticipates the speed and direction of the pitch and then aims his bat to bring it in line of the ball to hit it. Anticipation is predominant visual skill for the batter. Aiming follows it and is achieved by aligning with pitcher's hand, torso and his stance.

PITCHING

Pitching denotes the delivery of the ball to the batter. The pitcher throws the ball from the stationary position at the pitcher's plate using changes in ball speed and movement caused by air friction and spin to deceive the batter

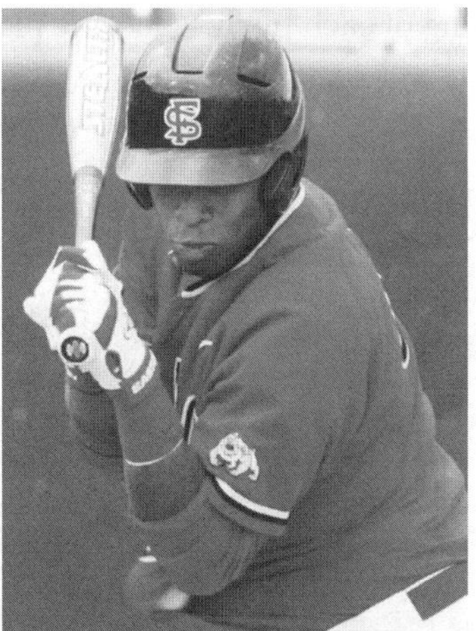

Fig. 14.2: Power hitting batting.

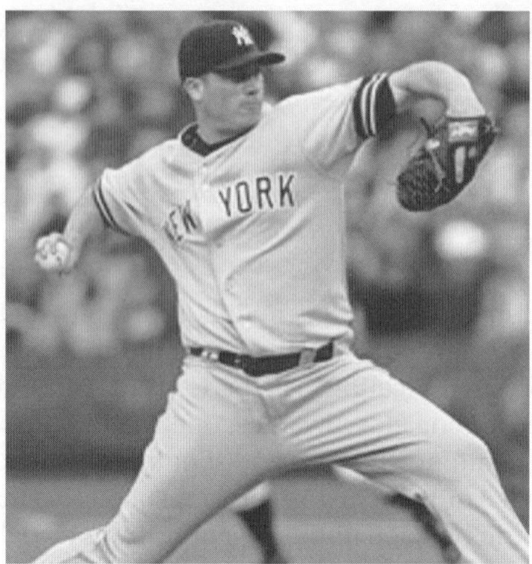

Fig. 14.3: Aiming to pitch.

(Fig. 14.3). The aim of pitching is to prevent the batter from scoring runs and getting them out. A single pitcher starts the game and makes every pitch until a point where the coach replaces tiring pitcher with a relief pitcher. The replaced pitcher cannot return to pitch again in the same game in normal course. Pitcher takes one step backward and one forward, to aim the ball at the batter. Aiming is achieved in accordance with the batter's stance.

FIELDING

Baseball is a lower scoring game which implies moments of poor pitching and individual fielding mistakes may prove very expensive. A player who is good batter, but not a competent fielder, may not play in the international games for long regularly. Baseball fielder must throw immediately after catching the ball **(Fig. 14.4)**. Only the pitcher's and the catcher's locations are fixed, and that only at the beginning of each pitch. Thus, the players on the field move

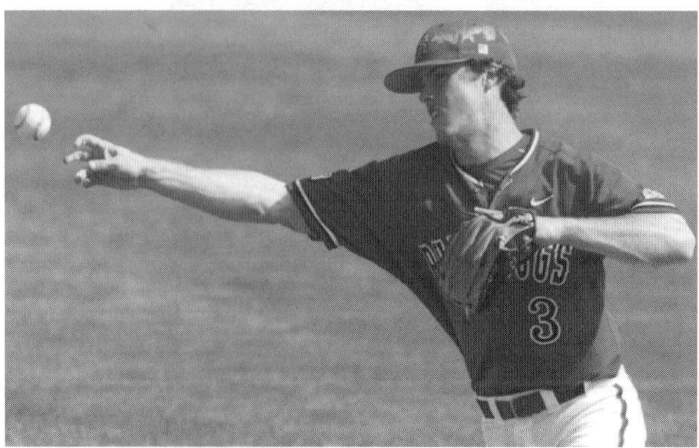

Fig. 14.4: Fielding in baseball.

around as needed to defend against scoring a run. Many variations of this are possible as locations depend upon situations. Whatever be the locations, the catcher anticipates the ball in air to aim his hands to catch the ball and then throw it. Anticipation dominates more than the aiming while fielding.

The importance of various elements of visual system in Baseball can be understood by following description:

VISUAL ACUITY

In baseball visual acuity is the most important visual skill to enhance the competitive edge. A baseball player requires an excellent visual acuity over a wide range of distances to improve his potential. For example, the batter must see the ball leaving the pitcher's hand at about 60 feet, or an outfielder must be able to focus on a fly ball that starts some 300 feet from him. Also, an infielder must see ground ball all the way into his glove. The importance of dynamic visual acuity is, therefore, more when referring to a batter trying to hit a pitched ball, an outfielder tracking the movement of a fly ball as he is running, and to a base runner trying to pick up any signals that a base coach may be giving him as he is running. Good contrast leads to enhance visual acuity. Color vision is not very important because of predetermined set of colors used for all accessories.

ACCOMMODATION–VERGENCE FUNCTION

A baseball player utilizes focus flexibility or vergence eye movements in baseball every time the baseball is moving. A baseball player must be able to focus at varieties of distances both far and near as the ball is moving towards them while they are batting and when they are running to chase a fly ball that has flown over the head. Focus flexibility allows a baseball player the ability to have clear, focused vision at all aspects of the game of the baseball.

OCULOMOTOR SKILL

In baseball saccadic eye movements, vestibular ocular movements and pursuits are all used in eye tracking. Saccades are used to scan a wide peripheral area and can be used to jump the eyes to a new fixation target. Vestibular eye movements are used to maintain fixation on an object during head movements when an outfielder is tracking a fly ball as he is running. Pursuit eye movements are used to track a moving baseball. However, fixation ability at the target is more important for the pitcher.

DEPTH PERCEPTION

Anticipation based on depth perception is the primary visual skill for the batter who anticipates the speed and direction of the ball in the air to hit. He needs to develop the spatial judgement of the ball so that he can time his shot correctly. Poor depth perception may lead to poor timing or missing the hit.

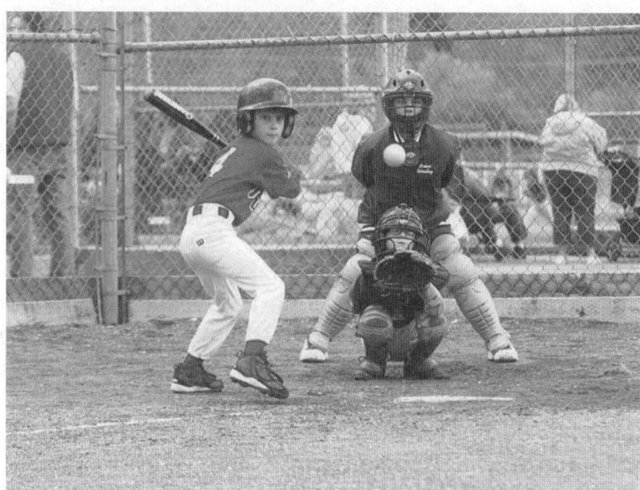

Fig. 14.5: Anticipating the speed and direction of the ball in the air to hit.

Therefore, the batter must judge where the ball comes from and where it is heading in order to calibrate the proper swing to hit the baseball **(Fig. 14.5)**. A fielder must use the same tactics to judge the position and eventual path of a batted ball. He must also judge the distance that they need to throw the baseball. Depth perception is not so critical while pitching the baseball which is predominantly an aiming activity.

■ BINOCULAR VISION

Good binocular vision is very important in baseball batting as the batter needs to be aware of his both sides to execute his shot effectively. Unless binocular vision is established early in the life, stereopsis cannot develop which affects catching ability while fielding and anticipating ability while batting. Besides, good binocular vision also enhances contrast and thereby visual acuity.

■ CENTRAL-PERIPHERAL AWARENESS

A baseball player must be aware of all of his surroundings at all times and be able to utilize his peripheral vision as a means to pick up objects such as a baseball, then be able to fixate on them. Take the instance of a batter, the batter knows the general beginning of where exactly a pitch may be coming from. The same is true for that of an outfielder. The general start of the ball is known, but exactly where is it going to drop is a question. The baseball must be recognized in the fielder's peripheral vision before a player can jump to it and fixate on it.

EYE-HANDS COORDINATION

The batter hits the ball with the bat held in the hands. He fixates on the center of the target, i.e., ball and moves his hand and eyes to search for the position before initiating motor movement of the arm or hand to hit the ball. So eye-hand coordination is not only very important in batting but it has to be very fast. Hard hitting nature of baseball makes eye-hand coordination a very important skill in baseball. While fielding eyes, hand, body and foot coordination becomes very important because if the fielder cannot balance himself while running towards the ball to pick it up or catch, he will not be able to aim at the target correctly.

GLARE RECOVERY

Since the baseball is played during the day, for the majority of its players, the importance of glare protection from sunlight cannot be over ruled. A player may wish to utilize tinted lenses when the sun can be blinding to a fielder. However, if the baseball is played under the stadium lighting, fast glare recovery becomes more important. The effect of glare tends to reduce the acuity and slows down the reaction time, creating a higher possibilities of injuries and resulting in poor performance.

In a study it has been seen that professional baseball players showed excellent ability to discriminate moving objects against various backgrounds. Compared to minor league players, they demonstrated higher stereopsis and contrast sensitivity. Also, a greater number of players in baseball have better visual acuity than 6/6. However, baseball is listed in the high risk categories for sports related eye injuries due to baseball being a hard and fast projectile. Younger players are more at risk because they could easily be hit by a pitched ball because of their poor skill and slow reaction time. Several organizations have developed a list of standards for protective eyewear equipment and other accessories used in baseball to ensure the safety. The most important property of the protective goggle is a strong polycarbonate lens with a durable and supportive frame design. Prescription devices in baseball may be designed with padding that fits comfortably and absorbs shock and provides cushioning effect.

Visual Demands in Golf

15 CHAPTER

TERMINOLOGIES

Ace, Eagle, Birdie, Par, Bogey, Double bogey, Fairway, Putting, Whiff, Knee knocker, Chip, Approach, Club, Pin, Hook, Slice

Golf is an outdoor sport played with a set of club and a small white ball over cross country course of eighteen holes. Each hole is separated by several hundred yards long distance with a fixed starting point. The object of the game is to complete the course which is several miles long, in as few strokes as possible. There are basically three types of shots—driving, approaching and putting mostly played in golf. The starting point is a flat ground on which the athlete "tee up" his ball on a small rubber peg or "tee". He, then hits the ball towards the hole, concentrating on achieving distance. From the tee to near the hole is the "fairway" which consists of fairly smooth ground but not entirely devoid of natural obstacles. The player continues to play towards the hole, concentrating mainly on direction. The actual hole is on the "green". The player covers the last few yards by the delicate art of "putting".

In the context of sports vision whether the game of golf should be considered dynamic or a controlled sport - has always been a matter of debate. Some people consider golf as fairly relaxing and "easy on the body" activity and therefore, consider it to be a sport of lazy people. In a controlled sport action of the event is normally repetitive and continues over many hours and important skill required is not just hitting the target once correctly and skillfully, but its consistency over the entire day. Golf is characterized by the slowness with regard to the speed of the game and the repetitive action of the three main shots, spread over many hours, which requires long-sustained skill to maintain consistency over the day. This may be the reason why they put golf into the category of controlled sport. But research shows that swinging a golf club is highly physical and neurological taxing event. In fact, hitting a golf shot requires the same amount of exertion on the body as lifting a weight that one can lift four times before having to rest. And the number of such strokes through the game is also not less. Even an amateur golfer can swing the ball at over 100 mph. About 90% of all their muscular strength is needed to execute it which is nowhere less than what is needed in football or hockey. Every joint in the body must rotate during a golf swing. Although golf does not require body building but really requires static and dynamic stabilization as well as inter-muscular coordination. This shows the explosiveness involved in the

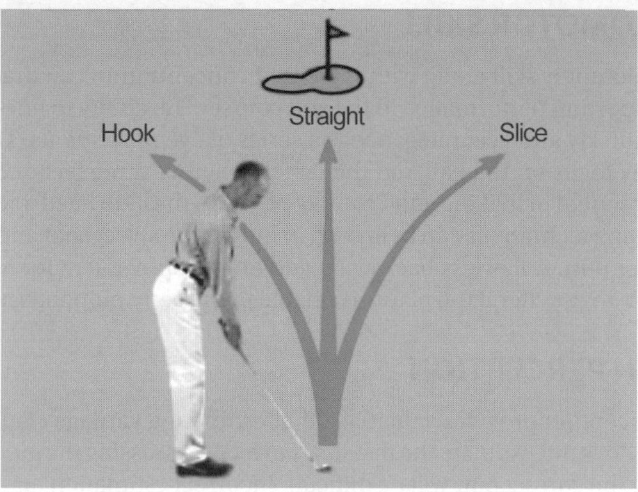

Fig. 15.1: Fixing the body posture to aim in golf.

golf, which puts it into the category of dynamic sport. In view of the above we may categorize golf as a dynamic sport which has some elements of controlled sport also.

Golf is an aiming sport in which anticipation is equally important. Aiming is needed to hit the ball from the teeing to fairway and also while making the putt. Whereas anticipation is needed to judge the distance between ball and the fairway and then between the ball and the hole while putting. In golf while hitting the ball there is no fixed alignment available to aim with. The golfer aims by aligning his body with general direction through the center of the fairway. Peripheral awareness becomes very important in this respect. Fixing the body posture in sideway stance helps hitting the ball at the aimed point **(Fig. 15.1)**.

The importance of various elements of visual system in Golf can be understood by following description:

VISUAL ACUITY

The game of golf consists of hitting a small ball with the club from the teeing ground to the green, where it is putted into a small round hole. Static visual acuity is more important than dynamic visual acuity. Good contrast is needed to hit the white ball. Color vision is not very critical.

ACCOMMODATION-VERGENCE FUNCTION

The predominance of aiming requires good convergence and divergence facility in golf and the ability to shift focus from near to distance effectively is particularly linked with putting performance.

OCULOMOTOR SKILL

Good oculomotor skill along with increased concentration can dramatically increase sporting performance in the golf course. The ability to fine-focus on a target, quickly and accurately needs a series of eye movements. The ability to properly focus on the ball and the target, whether three feet or 300 yards away, is essential in making good contact between the club head and the ball. Fine focusing techniques can help both in hitting the sweet spot and stroking a smoother putt. A flawless backswing and an uncanny talent for hitting the sweet spot, may suffer if the player is unable to properly pinpoint the target.

DEPTH PERCEPTION

Depth perception provides valuable aid in estimating yardage **(Fig. 15.2)**. If the golfer does not estimate the distance correctly, assessing the green as well as making the correct putt will be difficult. Incorrect estimation may lead to a situation where the golfer is constantly hitting the ball either short or too long or may be towards the left or right of the hole.

BINOCULAR VISION

Binocular vision is the predisposing factor for an elite class golfer. Binocular vision facilitates aiming especially in golf as there is no fixed alignment available. It also provides golfer good depth perception ability to judge distance and direction. Wider field of vision, better contrast are the other attributes of binocular vision that enhances visual performance and thereby improves sporting performance in golf. Strong dominant eye facing forward while hitting the ball is always more advantageous than using non-dominant eye for correct aiming and measuring the distance.

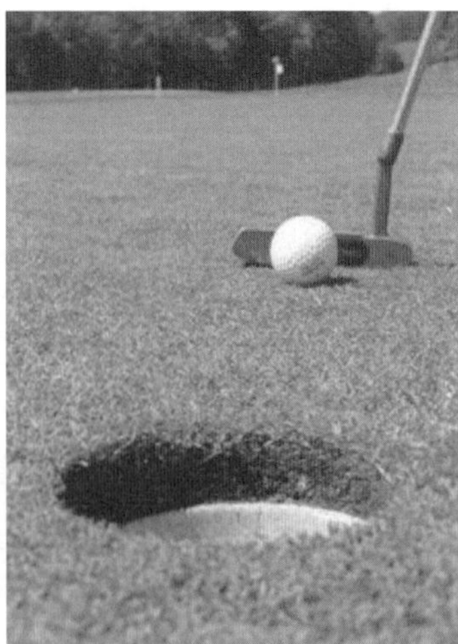

Fig. 15.2: Judging the distance between the ball and hole to putt.

CENTRAL-PERIPHERAL AWARENESS

Central-peripheral awareness is very critical visual skill in golf as aiming is achieved by aligning the body with general direction through the center of the fairway for which peripheral awareness is equally important. In this way central-peripheral awareness helps in both—aiming and anticipation. It also allows the player to be aware of the ball and at the same time being aware of where he wants to hit the ball.

EYE-HAND-BODY COORDINATION

Eye, hand and body coordination is probably the most important visual skill in golf **(Fig. 15.3)**. A golfer spends good amount of time in balancing his entire body before hitting the ball. The golfer needs to be comfortable and relaxed at stance. If the fundamentals of a good position are not present, the required chaining effects of movement cannot occur efficiently and effectively. Let's visualize a golfer tee off, he takes the sideways stance with legs apart and the club in his hand. The club appears to be an extension of his hands and arms as he begins the backswing head down, eyes on the ball, knees slightly flexed, arms firm. All muscles work in concert with one another, producing one fluid movement, as he makes the downswing, hitting the club head perfectly on the ball and continuing with his follow-through to complete the circle. This looks like a sequential step of a beautiful dancing and is a result of good eye-hand-body coordination. Hitting the ball hard requires keeping the body square to the target line and positioning the feet appropriately for the club you are going to use. The line of the tips of your toes, knees, hips, and shoulders should be parallel to your target line. All these are the essential qualities of a good golfer which is the function of good eye and body coordination.

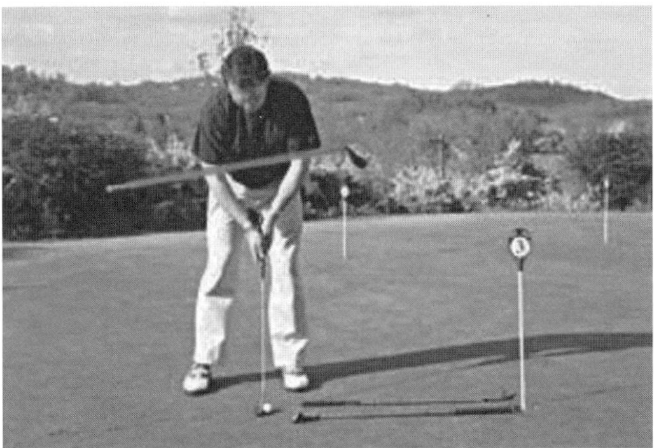

Fig. 15.3: Typical eye-hand-body coordination in golf.

GLARE RECOVERY

Glare disability can be a major problem on the golf course. Bright sunlight takes its toll on both the mental and physical aspects of performance and makes reading the green difficult. Reading the green accurately refers to the process of analyzing the slope, grain, and contours of the putting surface on a golf course. This helps golfers determine how a putt will break and fast the ball will roll. Glare can also be caused by annoying reflections from sands, water, etc. Fortunately, varieties of products in the form of sunglasses are available to protect the eyes from glare.

Golf is a slow moving sport and involves each participant taking turns. Surprisingly visual dynamics of golf are very essential elements for big success. Visualization are often useful in developing consistency in performance. Simply stated, if you can imagine yourself performing a proper swing often enough, you will tend to actually perform the swing in a like manner. So far safety is concerned ocular injuries in golf are not very common, but the golf ball has potential to produce serious eye injuries.

Visual Demands in Hockey

16 CHAPTER

TERMINOLOGIES

Hit, Flick, Push, Scoop, Dribbling, Jab, Lunge, Deke, Dig, Elbowing, Forward, Goal, Linesman, Offside, Penalty, Referee

Hockey is a dynamic team sport played outdoor with 11 players in each side, one of them is a goalkeeper. It is played with a wooden stick and a ball on a big ground with goal post at its both ends **(Fig. 16.1)**. The entire team wears an identical dress to provide an aesthetic brilliance to the game. The goalkeeper is only one who is allowed to use pads, gloves and front cover helmet for the safety. Hit, flick, push, scoop, dribbling, jab, lunge are the prominent strokes employed in the game. Physical fitness, supple wrist, quick reflexes, speed, agility and eagle eyes which may be innate or acquired are important qualities for a successful hockey player. But most important thing which differentiate between a good player and a great player is the ball control which is highly visually dependent. The team that has better ball control invariably carries the day. The first thing, of course, is to gain the possession of the ball, then the time of its release is equally important. A game of hockey consists of two 35 minutes playing periods, separated by a five-minute break. The team changes their halves after the break.

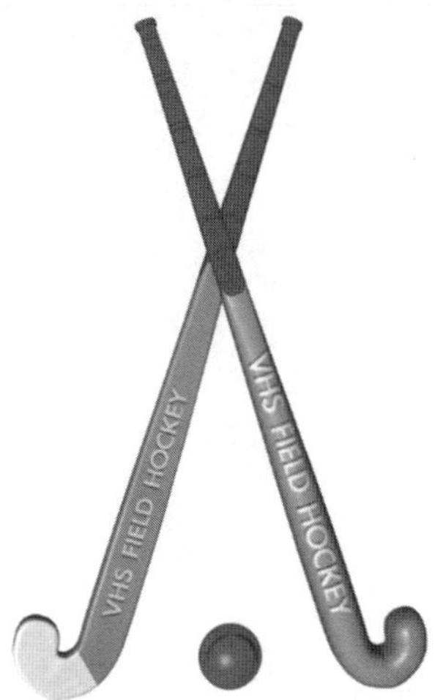

Fig. 16.1: Ball and stick in hockey.

The player needs to have a constant awareness of their spatial relationship to their teammates and the opponents and have to anticipate the speed and the direction of the ball to make his position to aim his stick to hit the ball. So it is predominantly an anticipatory sport. Even the goalkeeper anticipates the direction and the spatial location of the ball to fix up his position or aim his stick or legs to stop the ball. Aiming is, therefore, secondary and is achieved in relation to the position of the other player, his stick and the ball. But the visual characteristics of the goalkeeper is slightly different which certainly include anticipation through good depth perception and ability to aim in terms of knowing where the ball would be in relation to his stick and body. The goalkeeper needs great courage and confidence which is dependent on visual performance.

The importance of various elements of visual system in Hockey can be understood by following description:

VISUAL ACUITY

Dynamic visual acuity is more critical in hockey than static visual acuity because both the players and the ball are always in motion **(Fig. 16.2)**. It is because of its explosiveness with respect to speed. Good visual acuity is very critical because of small target size and speed. Good contrast acuity is also necessary because of the speed and poor contrast between the object and its ground. The importance of contrast sensitivity increases during fog or mist or during evening time. Color perception is not very important.

ACCOMMODATION–VERGENCE FUNCTION

The ability of the eyes to work in unison while tracking a moving ball and to change focus instantaneously as the distance of the ball changes in relationship

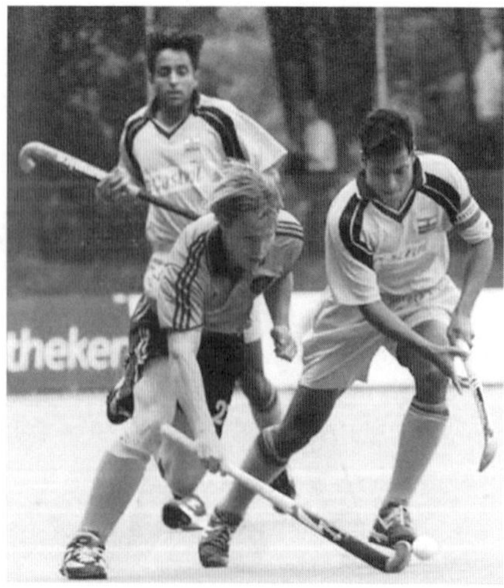

Fig. 16.2: Both players and the ball are in motion.

to your own position, is very important in hockey. For goalkeeper it is really very important to adjust the eyes rapidly over a great distance in order to keep an eye on the ball. It is a sport that requires quick vergence function.

OCULOMOTOR SKILL

Fixation is important skill for the goalkeeper during penalty shots and the player needs to have a momentary fixation when they aim to pass the ball to the fellow teammate or at the goal. The explosive nature of the sport requires full range of quick tracking ability to receive a pass or defend a goal.

DEPTH PERCEPTION

Since hockey is predominantly anticipatory sport, depth perception is a critical visual skill for the player and also for the goalie. Excellent depth perception allows him to judge the distance, speed and direction of the ball as it approaches the net **(Fig. 16.3)**. Players need to know where their teammates are in relation to the opposite team's players in order to make effective passes. In a one on one situation, good depth perception helps you judge when to make your move in relation to the defensive player between you and the net. Poor depth perception directly affects the anticipation skill which ultimately reduces performance at the competitive level.

BINOCULAR VISION

In hockey the players are scattered throughout the ground. The player who is moving with the ball needs to know the position of the teammates on his either side and also the position of the players of the opponent's team. Binocular vision is very critical. It also facilitates depth perception and enhances contrast and peripheral awareness. Binocular vision is also important while aiming at the goal post during the penalty shot.

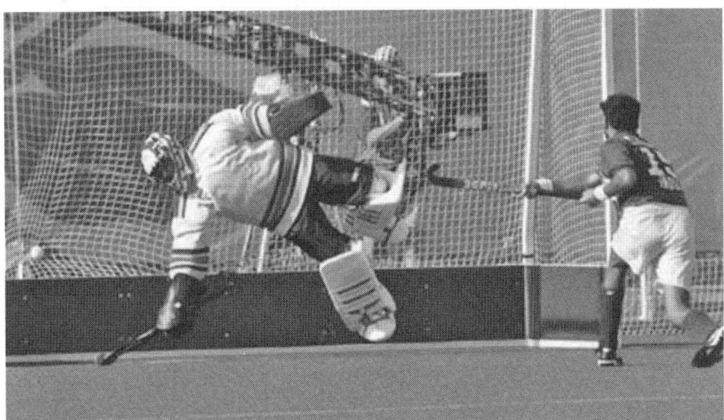

Fig. 16.3: Goalkeeper is anticipating the direction of the ball to defend.

■CENTRAL-PERIPHERAL AWARENESS

Central-peripheral awareness is also important visual skill needed to know the position of the opponents and the teammates and also to be aware of the goalkeeper position at the goalpost. Good central-peripheral awareness also facilitates anticipation and movement in between gaps.

■EYE-HAND COORDINATION

The process of taking a pass and accurately shooting to the open part of the net is one of the prime examples of this skill. Eye-hand coordination plays an important part in deflecting shots and knocking down high passes, or in helping a goalie to make a glove save.

■GLARE RECOVERY

Hockey is played outdoor in large grounds where players line of gaze direction and head orientation mostly denies the impact of glare on vision.

Hockey is highly visually demanding sport. With the explosive dynamics of 22 players accelerating and rapidly moving in all directions on the playing field, not only physical fitness is essential but also efficient visual system and quick visual reactions are necessary for the success. All position in hockey require good visual system. Ocular injuries are not much reported in hockey.

Visual Demands in Basketball

17 CHAPTER

TERMINOLOGIES

Assist, Bounce, Draft, Block, Chest pass, Basket, Dribble, Overhead pass, Possession, Baseline, Point guard

A traditional basketball team has 12 players, with five basketball players on the court at any given time. Unlimited substitutions are allowed. Basketball is a fast and dynamic sport played on a rectangular hard surface of 26 meters in length and 14 meters in width, measured from the inside edge of the boundary lines **(Fig. 17.1)**. The goal consists of posts that have iron rings and short nets attached to them and backboards. It is played with a ball resembling football. It is purely a handling game and the ball is advanced by dribbling, bouncing and passing. Advancing more than two steps with the ball in hand is not allowed. Deliberate body contact is not allowed. The aim of the game is simple—to score points by putting round ball into goal, known as basket and to prevent the opponent team from scoring. The game consists of two halves of 20 minutes each with an interval of 10 minutes. Basketball is a male-dominated sport, although female also plays. Heights of the players is considered the most important asset in addition to the long-sustained stamina.

In basketball, all the players are spread on the field and they look for the ball either from their teammate as a pass or try to steal away the ball from opponents and finally shoot it into the basket. During the process they keep

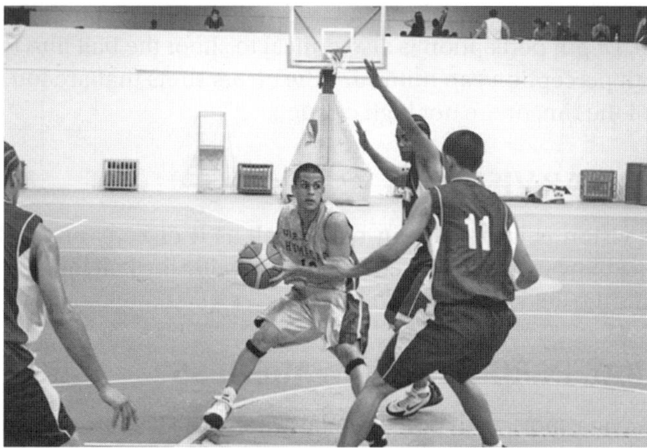

Fig. 17.1: Game of basketball.

the eyes on the spatial localization of the ball with the peripheral awareness of the other players. Anticipation is the predominant visual skill. Aiming is needed to shoot the ball into the basket or to pass to the teammate which is achieved by aligning with the desired target.

The importance of various elements of visual system in Basketball can be understood by following description:

VISUAL ACUITY

Basketball is a sport of almost constant motion, for the players and the ball, so well-developed dynamic acuity is just as significant as good static acuity. However, larger physical size of ball casts larger image on the retina. Vision may be affected by the position of the luminaries if the game is played indoors. Color vision and contrast acuity are not very critical in basketball.

ACCOMMODATION–VERGENCE FUNCTION

The players have to constantly and quickly shift his focus from near to far or intermediate targets throughout the contest. At times long-sustained accommodation vergence facility is needed in basketball.

OCULOMOTOR SKILL

Fixation is very essential to shoot the ball into the basket. Saccades are more important than pursuits. Quick, accurate saccades are important to survey the locations and movements of the ball and other nine players in relationship to the basket, boundary lines, etc.

DEPTH PERCEPTION

Depth perception helps to anticipate the position of opponents to steal away the ball from them, the position of teammates to pass the ball and also to judge the speed and direction of throw so as to ensure accurate pass **(Fig. 17.2)**. Depth perception is also critical to shoot the ball into the basket. Good depth perception can minimize the errors shots that are too long, that fall short of the rim, or are not high enough.

BINOCULAR VISION

Binocular vision is important in basketball as it directly affect the depth perception ability which is very critical for throwing the ball into the basket. It also extends the field of clear vision.

CENTRAL-PERIPHERAL AWARENESS

In a fast moving sport, with both the players and the ball in constant motion, knowing where you are, in relation to the position of teammates and players

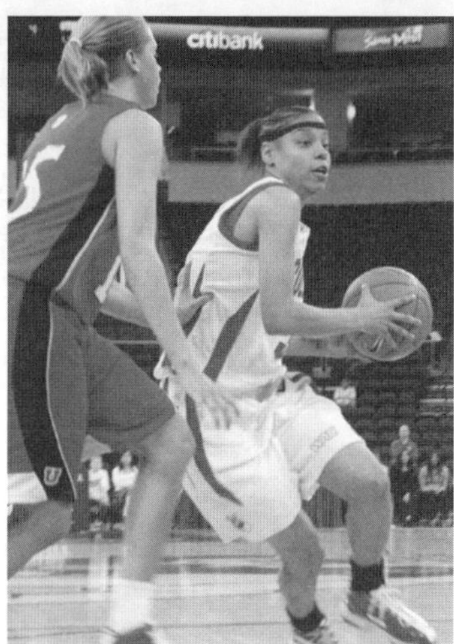

Fig. 17.2: Trying to steal away the ball.

of opposite team, the ball, other players, and the basket is very important. It facilitates making empty areas and hence reaching to the target and passing the ball to teammates.

EYE-HAND-BODY COORDINATION

The fast eye-hand coordination **(Fig. 17.3)** is definitely a great skill in basketball. Great basketball player does have great eye-body coordination also which can be seen when they catch a pass while running or slipping.

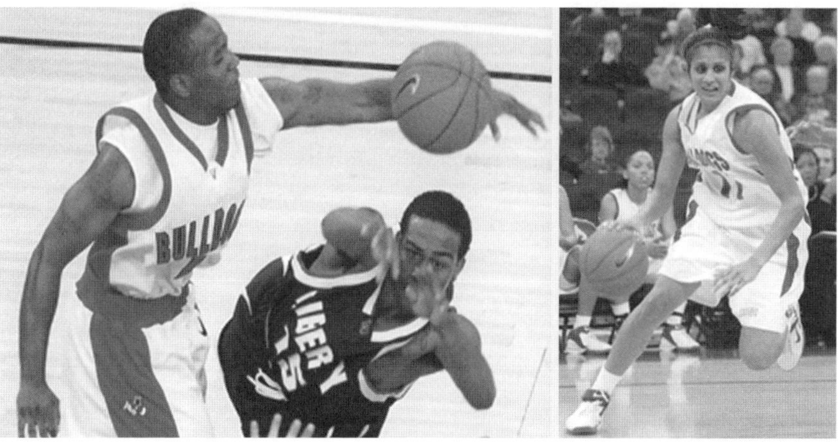

Fig. 17.3: Fast eye-hand-body coordination in basketball.

GLARE RECOVERY

Glare recovery is not very important in basketball as it is mostly played indoors in diffused lights.

The game of basketball is very fast where the players do not have time to think and visualize. Fast eyes and fast reaction are key to success. As far as ocular injuries are concerned, they are not much reported in basketball.

Visual Demands in Volleyball

18 CHAPTER

TERMINOLOGIES

Ace, Antenna, Approach, Assist, Attack, Beach dig, Block, Bump, Bump pass, Campfire, Cut shot, Decoy, Dig, Dink, Foul, Held ball, Joust

Volleyball is considered one of the fastest sport in the world. The speed, aggression and the agility of the players makes it a dynamic sport. Volleyball is played between the two teams of six players each **(Fig. 18.1)**. The object is to shed the ball over a net and within the boundaries of the court, so that the opposing team is unable to return or prevent it from hitting the ground. Basically there are two types of pass, the upper hand pass and the underhand pass. These can be executed from fixed position, in jump, after movement and also with body throw. The athletes may use one or both hands to perform. The game starts with a toss to decide either the end or the service. The winner of the toss decides to choose either the end or he prefers to serve first. All international matches are decided to the best of three or five sets. After each set the team changes the end, except when the following set is the decider. Ends of the court in the deciding set are chosen after the second toss.

Like tennis, volleyball is predominantly an anticipatory sport. The players anticipate the direction and the speed of the ball and accordingly jumps onto

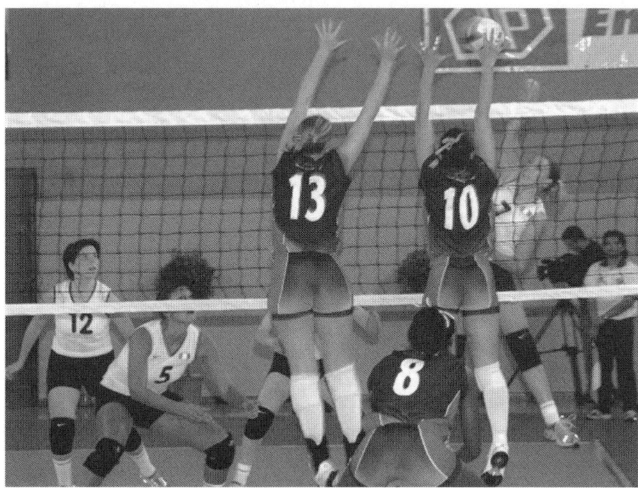

Fig. 18.1: Game of volleyball.

it or makes his position to bring his body and hands in line with the ball to return. Aiming follows the anticipation and is achieved with the position of the opponent, net and side poles of the net, keeping eyes onto the ball. During the serve also the player anticipates the gap or weak point in the opponent's court to aim his shot.

The importance of various elements of visual system in Volleyball can be understood by following description:

VISUAL ACUITY

Good eyesight is the foundation for all visual abilities. Every athlete should strive for optimum vision or better with or without correction. In fast moving volleyball, dynamic visual acuity is more important than static visual acuity **(Fig. 18.2)**. Color perception is not terribly critical to a volleyball player's performance as both teams stay on their own sides of the net. There is no need to sort out intermingled opponent player by the colors of their uniform. High contrast acuity is definitely advantageous in volleyball.

ACCOMMODATION–VERGENCE FUNCTION

This is also an important skill in volleyball because the ball and other players move quickly and one has to be able to shift focus from near to far or intermediate targets rapidly throughout the contest, while general body stamina is running down due to heavy exertion.

OCULOMOTOR SKILL

Fixation is somewhat important during serving process in volleyball. Otherwise it is not as critical as a skill to master as it is for archer or shooter. Knowing where you are in relation to the ball, the position of the other player

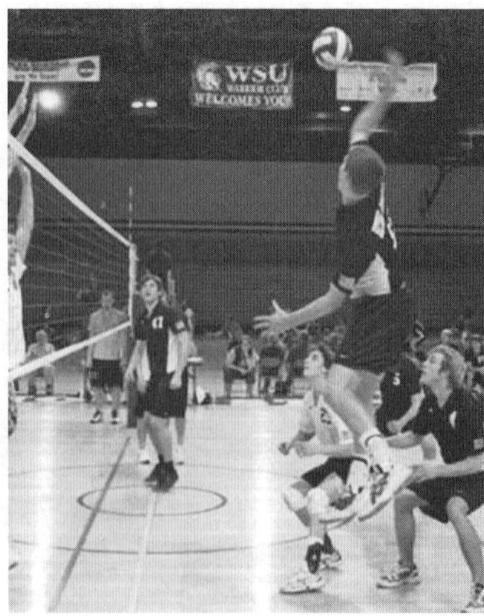

Fig. 18.2: Dynamic visual acuity and high contrast in volleyball.

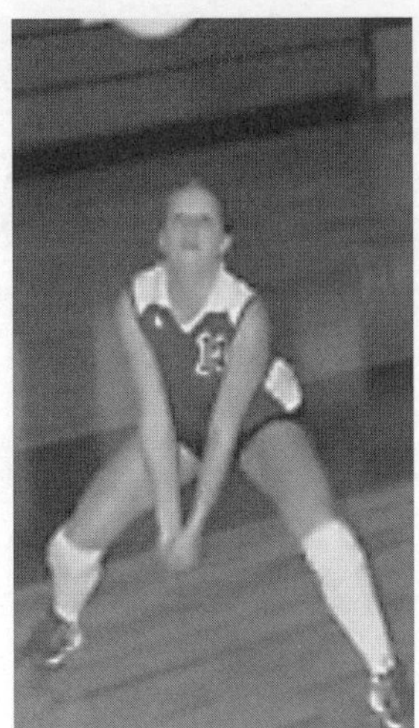

Fig. 18.3: Spatial localization of ball.

and opponents—all these require fast moving eyes. Quick, accurate saccades are needed for the purpose.

DEPTH PERCEPTION

Depth perception **(Fig. 18.3)** is very critical skill for volleyball player as it directly affects anticipation. This is very essential for accurate serving, setting and boundary line play, or no play decisions. It also enables a player to correctly perceive where the ball is in free space as well as other players.

BINOCULAR VISION

Good binocular vision adds to the visual skill as it improves peripheral awareness and depth perception which are important skills for volleyball player.

CENTRAL-PERIPHERAL AWARENESS

This is a very essential skill for superior performance in a game-like volleyball irrespective of his position on the ground. The player needs to know the position of his teammates and also the position of the opponent player while keeping his eyes on the ball. Peripheral awareness is also critical for no play decisions.

EYE-HAND-BODY COORDINATION

Throwing of body onto the ball, stretching hands to hit the ball, moving back while keeping the eyes on the ball in front—all these are the result of faster body reaction and accurate eye-hand-body coordination

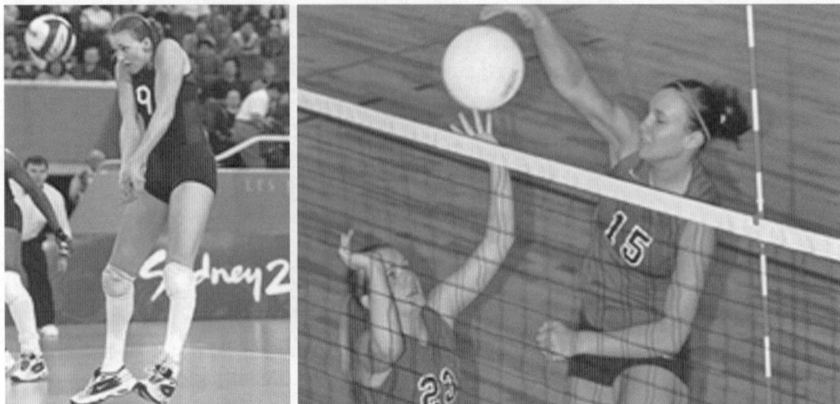

Fig. 18.4: Eye-hand-body coordination at the back and on the net.

(Fig. 18.4). In volleyball, all of these skills, especially eye-hand coordination, are essential for effective performance. During the overhand serve, being able to arm toss the ball precisely so that it falls to the spot just inside of the lead foot and in-line with the hitting shoulder, guiding the hand so that it follows the ball to the target, and finishing with the hand alongside or within the bodyline—necessitates extreme amount of eye-hand-body coordination.

GLARE RECOVERY

Glare recovery is important in volleyball due to the bright lighting in gymnasiums and sports arenas, especially during televised games when television crews bring additional spotlighting equipment.

Volleyball is a diving, leaping, net and ball team sport which caught the world around the World War II, is a visually demanding sport. One team serves the ball and the other returns and during this process they need good eyesight. About ocular injuries, they are not much reported in this sport.

Visual Demands in Football

19 CHAPTER

TERMINOLOGIES

Bicycle kick, Corner flag, Corner kick, Cross, Defender, Free kick, Dribble, Off-side, Penalty, Penalty shot

Football is a fast-paced dynamic sport, played in an outdoor environment. It is a sport played between two teams, each consisting of 11 players, including one goalkeeper. It is played on a rectangular field having a length not more than 130 yards and breadth not more than 100 yards. At the two ends of the field there are two goalposts. The game starts by the choice of end or the kick-off, which is decided by toss. The game is officiated by a referee and two linesmen who enforce the law as applicable. The duration of the game is 90 minutes of two equal halves of 45 minutes each, unless otherwise mutually agreed upon. The result of the match is decided by the number of goals scored by the teams.

The object of the game is to score by maneuvering the ball into the opposing goal using feet. Occasionally, players also use their torso or head to propel the ball. No ball except the goalkeeper is allowed to use their hands or arms. The team that scores the most goals by the end of the match wins. If the score is tied at the end of the game, either a draw is declared or the game goes into extra time and/or a penalty shootout, depending on the format of the competition.

Goalkeeping is a specialized position in football and is very vital for building up a strong team. The cardinal principle of goalkeeping is "safety first". Both hands should be used and whenever possible, the goalkeeper should place his body behind his hands to form a second barrier to the ball. For a successful performance, a goalkeeper must develop other important skills like catching, throwing, fisting, diving for the ball and covering it together with stance. Balancing while kicking, trapping, passing, dribbling, heading, throwing, tackling and charging are the main skills of all other players.

Football is highly visually demanding sport. Anticipation based on depth perception is the predominant primary visual skill. The player anticipates the ball during the play and accordingly position himself to hit at the target. Aiming, therefore, is secondary and is achieved in relation to the position of the other player and the ball. However, the visual characteristics of the goalkeeper is slightly different which certainly include anticipation through good depth perception, and the ability to aim in terms of knowing where the ball would be in relation to his catching hands. The goalkeeper needs great courage and confidence, which is highly dependent on visual performance.

The importance of various elements of visual system in Football can be understood by following description:

VISUAL ACUITY

Football is a highly explosive team game. Basic tasks in football include kicking, throwing, passing, dribbling, heading, tackling and punting the ball. Good visual acuity is recommended for all position for spatial localization, anticipation timing, reactivity and confidence. Players must be able to see the ball on the move and measure the accuracy of aim. Dynamic visual acuity is more important than the static visual acuity as either the ball or the player is always in the motion **(Fig. 19.1)**. Good contrast is necessary for quick identification and tracking of the fast moving ball against various backgrounds. The need of high contrast increases when the football is played in mist and fogged weather. Good visual acuity is more critical for goalkeeper because any residual uncorrected refractive error might lead to missing of long balls and thereby loss of confidence while diving for the ball.

ACCOMMODATION–VERGENCE FUNCTION

Tracking the football, looking for the opponents and the teammates and finally receiving the ball on the toes and then hitting it, all of the activities are beyond the distance of near vision distance, accommodation and convergence are not very significant visual skills in football.

OCULOMOTOR SKILL

Football is highly explosive game. Full range smooth pursuits, and accurate saccadic eye movements are important in receiving a pass, identifying the

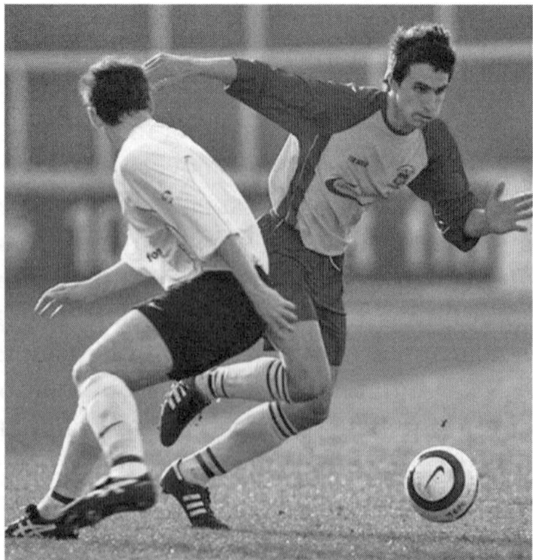

Fig. 19.1: Dynamic visual acuity in football.

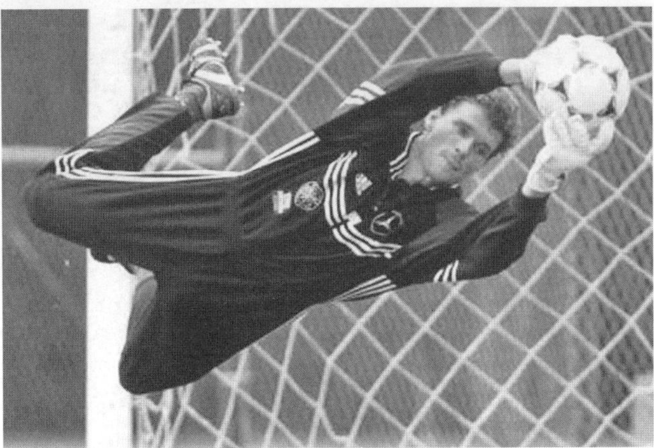

Fig. 19.2: Spatial judgement of ball.

open teammate and also catching the ball for the goalkeeper. At times during penalty shots fixation ability also becomes important.

DEPTH PERCEPTION

Depth perception is very critical for all position in football. The spatial position of ball, efficient and accurate perception of speed and direction of ball trajectory determines the timing for eye-hand-body-foot response. The ability to pass the ball out of the reach of a defender and into the goalpost is an example of depth perception skill in football. At times the player needs to anticipate the ball in the air and makes his position accordingly to receive it **(Fig. 19.2)**.

BINOCULAR VISION

Binocular vision provides **(Fig. 19.3)** an advantage of larger field of vision than the monocular vision. Since football is a team game, where players are widespread on a big ground and is characterized by short, long and high tossed shots, binocular vision is very critical. Anticipation, based on depth perception is directly affected by the binocular vision.

CENTRAL-PERIPHERAL AWARENESS

Positional relationship between teammates and opponents, finding the open receiver to pass the ball, maintaining the awareness of lines while running from sides, awareness of goalkeeper's position—all these necessitate the demand for peripheral vision. The skill is necessary not only for distance performance but also at near to avoid collision. Defensive backs often use central or foveal vision to watch the attacker while relying on peripheral awareness to monitor the pattern of attack **(Fig. 19.4)**. Often central-peripheral awareness in football is considered to be more important than good visual acuity.

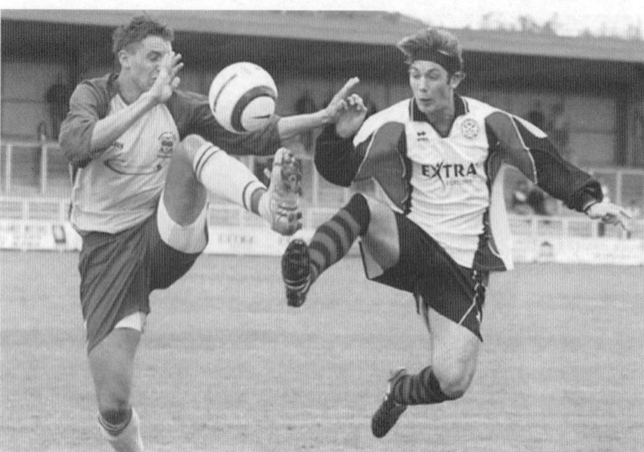

Fig. 19.3: Binocular vision is critical.

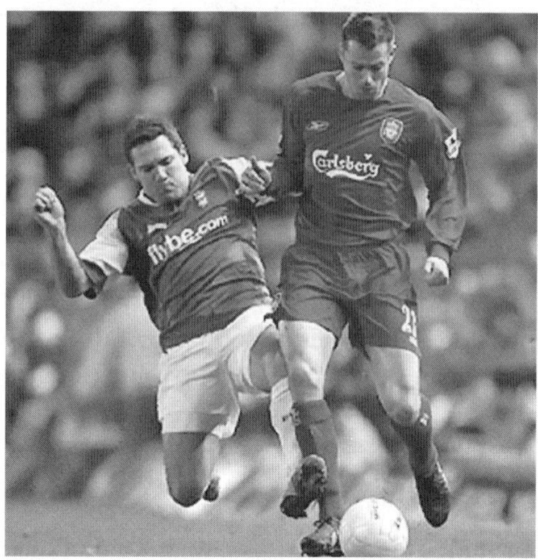

Fig. 19.4: Watching the ball and also aware of the attack from the sides by opponent.

■ EYE-HAND-FOOT-BODY COORDINATION

In football, all the players at positions require good eye, foot, body and hand co-ordination rather than just eye-hand coordination. Eye-hand co-ordination is particularly more important for the goalkeeper as he must look the ball into his hands with full body behind it. A fast, controlled coordination among eye-body-hand-foot is essential because of it explosiveness **(Fig. 19.5)**. A little delay during a pass may allow the gap to be filled. Similarly, a little delay on the part of goalkeeper to bring his hand or body behind the ball may cost the entire match. Eye-hand coordination is a function of the two primary components of visual performance—aiming and anticipation.

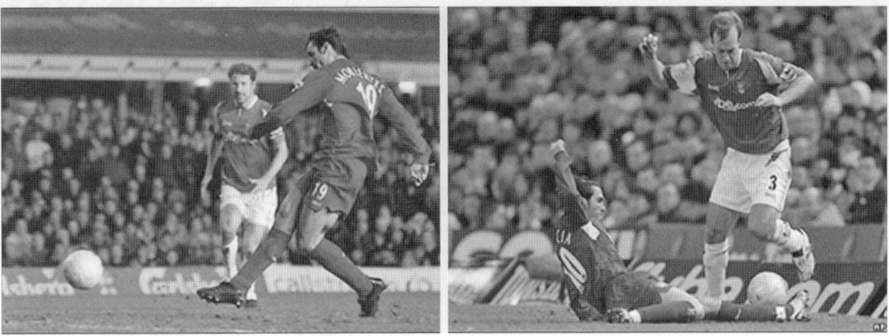

Fig. 19.5: Eye-foot coordination in football.

GLARE RECOVERY

Glare is not a critical factor in football. Only time when it can matter is the time when the goalkeeper is aiming to receive a penalty shoot and his eyes are dazzled because of some malpractice from the public.

With the explosive dynamics of 22 players accelerating and rapidly moving in all directions on the playing field, not only physical fitness is essential but also efficient visual system and quick visual reactions are necessary for the success. If you increase the speed at which an athlete perceives and responds to the stimulus, you decrease the duration of his reflex and thereby improves his performance. That sets for the fact that the football is highly visually demanding sport. All positions in football require good visual system with the highly-skilled jobs demanding more.

Visual Demands in Judo

20 CHAPTER

TERMINOLOGIES

Judoka, Judogi, Yuko, Dojo, Sensei, Zori, Ippon, Kata, Matte, Belt, etc.

Judo is an event of bare-handed fighting between two persons, played on a square of 8M × 8M mat. The sport emphasizes moral, intellectual training as well as physical training. It is a competitive and relaxing sport that is incidentally used as self-defense. The main objective of the sport is attainment of strength, health and utility by means of spiritual, moral and mental training. In spite of being a combat sport, discipline and control are the main essence of the sport and the main feature of the fight is the attainment of maximum results with minimum amount of energy expenditure. The sport lasts for a very short span of time and the winner is the athlete who scores more points at the completion of the time. A contest usually lasts for 3 to 10 minutes. The most important skill in Judo is the art of falling. Others include throw and grappling. Each throw consists of a series of steps in the sequence of unbalancing, moving into the position and actual throw. The sport comprises the elements of both dynamic sport as well as controlled sport.

The player must maintain perfect balance at all times because the moment the balance is broken; the opponent can throw him. The head is an important part of balance; the direction in which he faces is the direction of balance. The way the body is moved is also an important part of balance. He must keep the feet close to the mat at all times and walk erect. This suggests that aiming is an important skill in judo which may be achieved by opponent's position and his own body stance. Aiming is also needed to hit the opponent at the targeted point. Anticipation is equally important as it is needed to judge the opponent's reaction and also to reach to the targeted point while attacking.

The importance of various elements of visual system in Judo can be understood by following description:

VISUAL ACUITY

Judo is usually played in good lighting, where the target size is big and is characterized by comparatively less speed, all these reduces the demand for visual acuity **(Fig. 20.1)**. However, both static and dynamic visual acuity provide the additional edge to the athlete to make accurate judgment of the distance of the opponent before kicking or throwing. Contrast and color perception are of little or no importance.

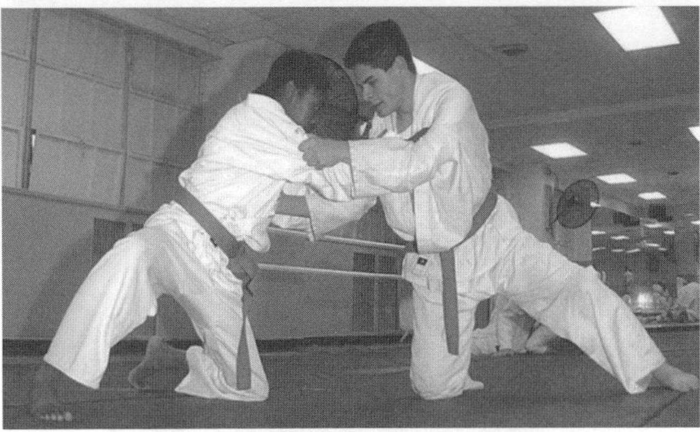

Fig. 20.1: Visual acuity in indoor judo.

ACCOMMODATION–VERGENCE FUNCTION

The player constantly focuses on the opponent's eyes, so focus flexibility is not very critical. Long-sustained vergence facility is also not very important as the judo is short duration sport.

OCULOMOTOR SKILL

Fixation ability is very critical in judo as the player constantly keeps his eyes on the opponent's eyes. The entire body balance right from the head to the feet is an integral part of the successful execution of attacks and defense in judo.

DEPTH PERCEPTION

Depth perception is very important in judo to anticipate the correct distance of the opponent and to kick or hold him effectively. Poor depth perception may result in week hold or ineffective kick, thereby affecting the performance. It also facilitates the ability to judge the opponent's attack.

BINOCULAR VISION

In judo, opponents can attack from both sides, making good binocular vision essential **(Fig. 20.2)**. Binocular vision also enhances peripheral awareness, which is critical in judo.

CENTRAL-PERIPHERAL AWARENESS

Central-peripheral awareness is an advantage that a sighted judoka enjoys over a visually impaired judoka. The sighted judoka gets the advantage of being aware of the relative position of himself and the opponent's position, that enables him to kick and throw successfully and also react fast enough to save the opponent's attack. In judo, peripheral awareness affects both aiming

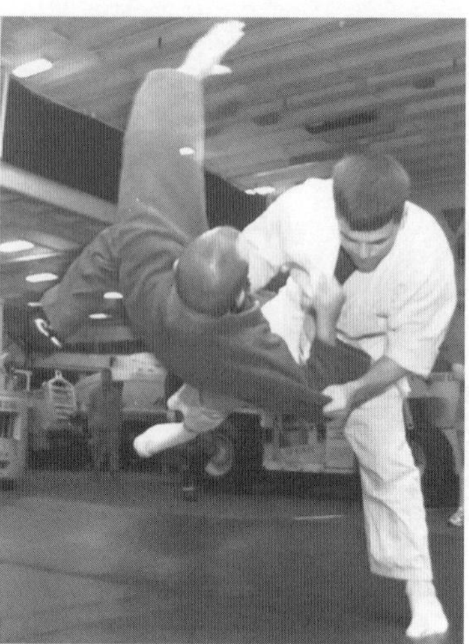

Fig. 20.2: Binocular vision in judo.

and anticipation. The spatial localization enables the athlete to plan, attempt and successfully make the desired move to obtain the desired result.

EYE-HAND-BODY COORDINATION

The fast reaction is the key to success in judo which makes eye-hand-body coordination an important factor. Judo player spend a large percentage of their time grappling with their opponent. The goal is to manipulate an opponent's body in order to take or throw him to the ground. Another important skill required is the ability to drive block and move the opponent behind **(Fig. 20.3)**. Judo players at the elite level develops strong eye-hand-body coordination.

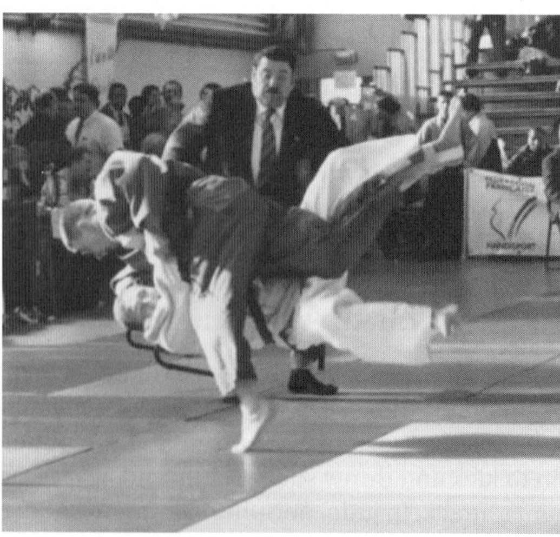

Fig. 20.3: Grappling with opponent.

That is why this sport is many a times used as an exercise to develop this skill in the sport like football or others where eye-hand-body coordination is needed. Eyes are also the important source of cue to understand the next move of the opponent.

GLARE RECOVERY

It is of less importance in judo, since it is an indoor sport with proper illumination facility and the player hardly look anywhere other than the opponent's eyes during the competition.

Judo is a highly explosive game in which addition to vision, past experience combined with good visualization techniques can help the athlete tremendously. Recalling, after a bad fight, what the opponent was doing to get through your defenses can enable a good athlete to adjust properly and quickly to close down the vulnerability, which may change the outcome of the repeat match between the same opponents. As far as ocular injuries are concerned, the most common are foreign body in the eyes, superficial injuries to eyelids, abrasion of lids, cornea and conjunctiva, contusion of eyeball and surrounding tissues.

Visual Demands in Wrestling

21 CHAPTER

TERMINOLOGIES

Round, Whizzer, Freestyle, Lift, Weight class, Headlock, Sprawl

Wrestling is the act of physical engagement between two unarmed persons. It is a combat sport played on a mat between two contestants, in which each wrestler strives to get an advantage over or control of the opponent. The physical activity which embody the style of wrestling are clinching, holding, locking and leverage. Modern professional wrestling is like an art which requires skill and proper training. Tremendous amount of agility, balance, strength and quick reaction skills are essential for a successful wrestler. The aggression, power and strength involved in the sport make it highly dynamic sport with good physical control. Wrestling is not a visually intensive sport. Aiming is needed only to get the hold to the targeted portion of the opponent's body while anticipation by depth perception is needed to the extent of arm's length and aiming is needed.

The importance of various elements of visual system in Wrestling can be understood by following description:

VISUAL ACUITY

Unlike other sports, big target size, bright light environment and the relatively slow speed of the target as well as of the athlete make it a less visually demanding sport **(Fig. 21.1)**. However, good static visual acuity enables the wrestler to read the scoreboard or the time remaining and accurately judge the distance of the opponent's leg before a takedown attempt. Contrast and colors perception are of little or no importance.

ACCOMMODATION–VERGENCE FUNCTION

There is almost no demand for accommodative facility beyond 40 cm. Also precise focusing is not of great importance as long as it does not affect visual acuity.

OCULOMOTOR SKILL

The entire body balance right from the head to the feet is an integral part of the successful execution of attacks and defense in wrestling. Eye motility must not

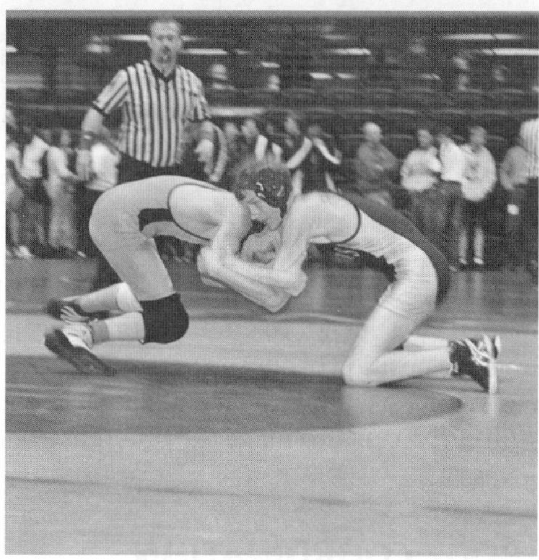

Fig. 21.1: Bright indoor light and big target size in wrestling.

be impaired during the bout. At times the wrestler does not have the choice or control of his head position and this is the time when eye motility becomes very critical for visual information. Fixation is pretty critical for accurate attack onto the opponent to score points.

DEPTH PERCEPTION

Depth perception ability is important only to the extent of the arm's length, as the target outside this distance is too far to reach **(Fig. 21.2)**.

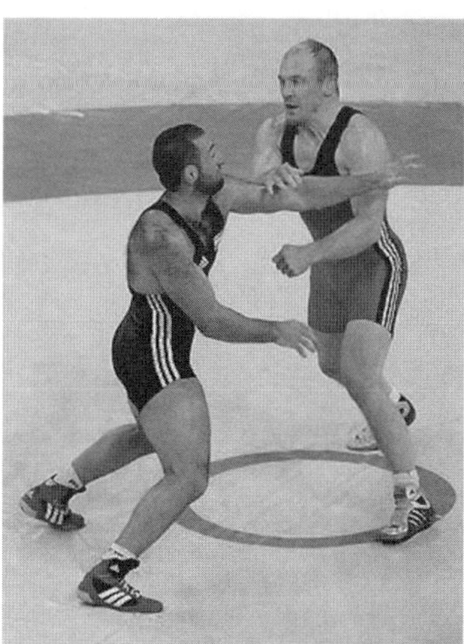

Fig. 21.2: Depth perception is important only to the extent of the arm's length.

BINOCULAR VISION

The wrestler attacks the opponent from both sides, therefore, good binocular vision is important in wrestling. Good binocular vision improves peripheral awareness which is very important for a wrestler.

CENTRAL-PERIPHERAL AWARENESS

Central-peripheral awareness is the chief advantage that a sighted wrestler has over a visually impaired wrestler. More than any other visual skill, the ability to be aware of the relative position of oneself and opponent's full anatomy can allow the wrestler to maintain control the fight to achieve successful end. The sense of spatial localization can also make the difference between attempted and completed moves.

EYE-HAND-BODY COORDINATION

The wrestler has to integrate a sense of balance with the visual-motor system **(Fig. 21.3)**. Wrestling is a fast sport, therefore in order for the fast reaction to be effective in the competition needs a high degree of eye-hand-body coordination. The exact time to stretch the hands, time to bring the body down to hold from the legs and constant front push of the body—all these are very critical in wrestling.

GLARE RECOVERY

Glare recovery of minor consideration due to bright light in and around the wrestling area and also because of flash photography. This is especially true

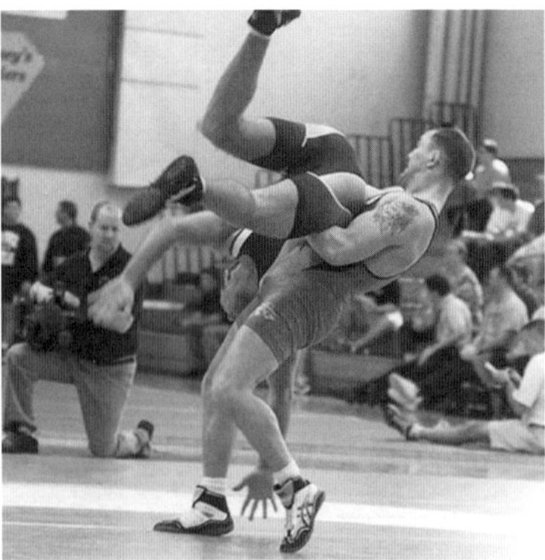

Fig. 21.3: Integrating a sense of balance with the visual-motor system.

during telecast bouts due to the extra lighting necessary for the television cameras. If the wrestler cannot recover quickly enough from a photographer's flash that catches him just before the opponent's attack, he may get knocked down in that split second of vulnerability.

Wrestling is a highly explosive game in which in addition to vision, past experience combined with good visualization techniques can help the wrestler tremendously. Recalling, after a bad match, what the opponent was doing to get through your defenses can enable a good wrestler to adjust properly and quickly to close down the vulnerability, which may change the outcome of the repeat match between the same opponents.

Visual Demands in Boxing

22 CHAPTER

TERMINOLOGIES

Jab, Hook, Uppercut, Cross, Punch, Counterpunch, Bob, Weave, Parry, Block, Clinch, Fist, Knockdown, Knockout

Boxing is an explosive, dynamic and power sport, characterized by punch, blow and hits. Two fighters of similar weight, fight within a ring. The game continues in a set of rounds of 3 minutes each. The victory is achieved when one of the fighters is able to knock the other down and who is unable to get up till the referee counts 3. Good boxer must be strong physically, quick in reaction, and skillful. He should also have courage and determination to play the cruel game of boxing in spite of pain and exhaustion. The boxer wears glove in his hands, a protection guard in his jaws, a half helmet on his head and a plastic cup to protect the groin area.

Before the game starts, the boxer adopts a basic stance in the ring, that helps sighting towards his opponent and stands with his feet apart allowing him easy and quick motion. He keeps his elbow close to his body to protect the ribs. Many left handed boxer adopt the same stance, though some of them may reverse it. The basic stance puts the boxer in the best position to avoid or block the punches of his opponents. The straight forward understanding is; anticipation predominates aiming in boxing **(Fig. 22.1)**. The boxer anticipates the speed and direction of opponents punch to save himself and then aims at him to hit with his counter punch. Aiming is achieved with an alignment of his opponent's eyes with the peripheral awareness of torso. Even while aiming to hit, anticipation becomes critical to judge the exact distance of the opponent so that he can hit him with full blow and power.

The importance of various elements of visual system in Boxing can be understood by following description:

■ VISUAL ACUITY

Tucked chin, lead shoulder slightly shrugged, elbows in, hands up, knees slightly bent, feet shoulder width apart, eyes wide open and staring at the opponent's eyes, all these pretending a posture of a tiger who is ready to attack his prey indicates the importance of good visual acuity in boxing **(Fig. 22.2)**. Boxing is a highly visually demanding sport where both static and dynamic visual acuity are important. Contrast may not be very critical as long as visual

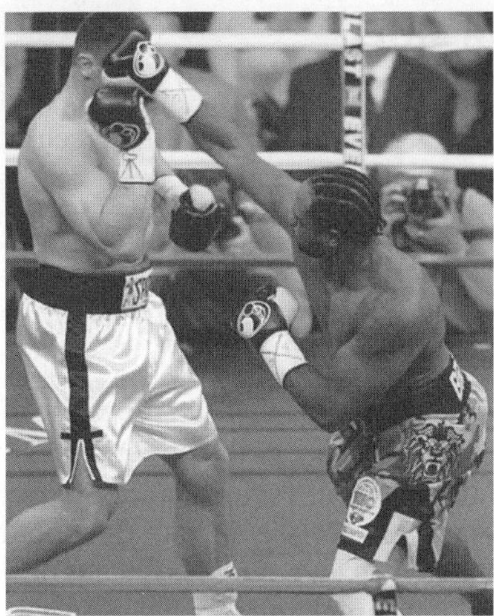

Fig. 22.1: Anticipation becomes critical to judge the exact distance of the opponent to hit with full blow and power.

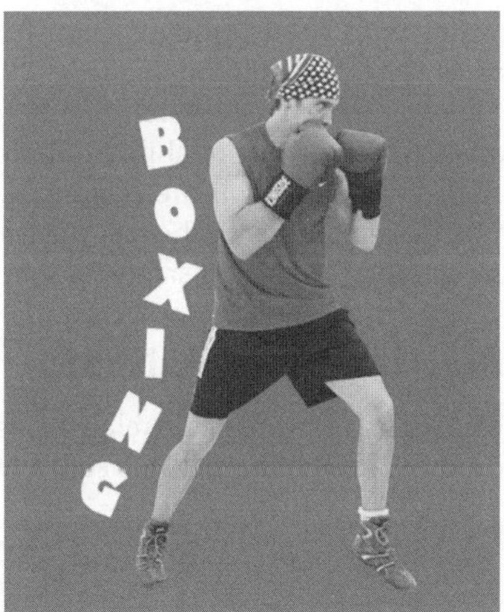

Fig. 22.2: Typical boxing posture, pretending to be tiger who is ready to attack his prey.

acuity is good enough as it is played in good illuminated indoor stadium. Color perception is also not very critical. The good visual acuity is very critical because of the speed of the punch and quick reactions.

ACCOMMODATION-VERGENCE FUNCTION

Accommodation and vergence function is not very critical in boxing because the entire fight is usually within five feet distance and the focus is constant on the opponent.

OCULOMOTOR SKILL

Fixation, saccades and eye tracking ability—all are very important oculomotor skills for boxing. Fixation is pretty critical for accurate landing of blows, quick and accurate saccades are needed to fixate on the moving opponent's vulnerable areas. Eye tracking ability is important for the boxer to hit the opponent who is constantly moving in front and around the ring.

DEPTH PERCEPTION

Depth perception is critical in boxing within the range of an arm's length. The boxer needs to judge exact distance of the opponent to hit him with full force. A blow administered by a boxer involves a snapping and twisting motion for which exact determination of the distance of the opponent is necessary for the blow to be most effective. It is also very critical to anticipate the speed and direction of the opponent's punch to make a good save.

BINOCULAR VISION

One boxer attacks other with hard punches from both sides, therefore, good binocular vision is very critical in boxing **(Fig. 22.3)**. Good binocular vision improves peripheral awareness which facilitates anticipation and also develops stereopsis which gives the ability to perceive depth to make the punch hard enough to knock down the opponent. The importance of binocular vision can be understood with the fact that monocular boxers are not allowed to play the game of boxing for safety reason.

CENTRAL-PERIPHERAL AWARENESS

It is important for the boxer to be aware of the relative positions of himself, his opponent, and surrounding environment. This sense of spatial localization

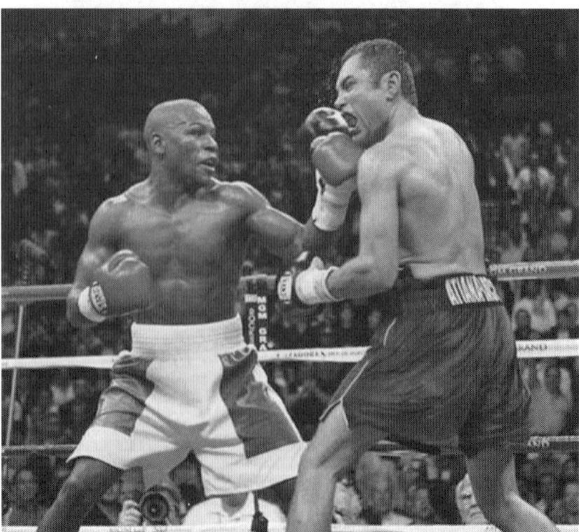

Fig. 22.3: Good binocular vision is very critical in boxing.

can make the difference between attempted and completed moves. In fact, peripheral awareness is very important in boxing which is hindered because of soft leather helmets used for safety reasons. It is an essential requisite for perfect anticipation.

EYE-HAND-BODY COORDINATION

The boxer has to integrate a sense of balance with the visual-motor system. Boxing is typically a very fast and quick reaction sport which necessitates a very high degree of eye-hand-body coordination. The exact time to stretch the hands, time to bring the body back and constant jump on feet—all these are very critical in boxing.

GLARE RECOVERY

Glare recovery is also one of the considerations due to bright light in and around the ring and also because of flash photography. This is especially true during telecast bouts due to the extra lighting necessary for the TV cameras. If the boxer cannot recover quickly enough from a photographer's flash that catches the boxer just right, he may get knocked out in that split second of vulnerability.

Boxing is a highly explosive game in which in addition to vision, past experience combined with good visualization techniques can help the boxer tremendously. Recalling, after a bad round, what the opponent was doing to get through his defenses can enable a good boxer to adjust properly and quickly to reduce the vulnerability. This is also highly exposed to injuries. Injuries in and around eye is quite common in boxing.

Visual Demands in Yachting

23 CHAPTER

TERMINOLOGIES

Abaft, Aft, Ahead, Apparent wind, Backing wind, Beam, Belayed, Bilge, Cleat, Draft, Leeway, Luffing, Mast, Squall

Yachting is a sport in which athletes race against each other on river, lakes, or on the ocean, depending upon the type of the race and discipline **(Fig. 23.1)**. The boats are propelled by the reaction forces on the oar blades as they are pushed against the water. The sport is highly competitive where overall fitness plays a large role. While sailing, one, two, four or eight athletes sit in the boat facing backwards, and uses the oars which are held in place by the oarlocks to propel the boat forward. The sport has a very high energy demand requiring lots of physical strength and endurance. The sport is characterized by both dynamic and control elements in almost equal proportion, with explosiveness being more dominating. Although the visual demand in yachting is not significant, the environmental conditions make it very important. The sailor relies on the wind pattern. The patterns of the wind on the water provides clues to its direction and intensity. He also relies on its sensation across the face and eyes to make tactical decisions in the race. Aiming and anticipation- both are needed in equal proportion. Aiming is mainly peripheral, using the banks of the river or lane markers as a reference. The general direction comes

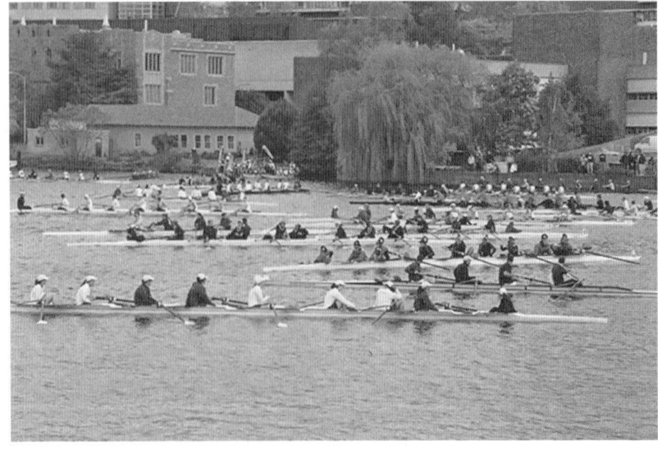

Fig. 23.1: Yachting.

from a marker buoy often at a great distance. Anticipation or depth perception is critical to the timing of the stroke and the rhythm of the crew.

The importance of various elements of visual system in Yachting can be understood by following description:

VISUAL ACUITY

Both static and dynamic visual acuity are important, due to the need to discriminate fine details while looking for markers, wind pattern on the surface of the water, other boats in the distance, etc. Although it is not a very fast moving sport, dynamic visual acuity may become important in foul weather and other extreme conditions. Contrast may not be very important except during the foul weather. Color perception is needed to discriminate color flags and other markers. Precipitation and wind speed, and reflection of the sunlight off the water surface may affect visual acuity.

ACCOMMODATION–VERGENCE FUNCTION

Fine judgement of relative speed and distance is needed when dipping behind other boats and for that there is a constant rapid adjustment from distance to near. Although there is no time to look at the competitor rowers directly and this is judged entirely by peripheral vision, in fierce competition, ocular fatigue may become a problem in the later stages of the race where there is convergence weakness.

OCULOMOTOR SKILL

In yachting, the yacht men propel the boat in a rhythm with the eyes mainly on buoy, navigational signals and other competitors by peripheral awareness, because of which eye movement is negligible.

DEPTH PERCEPTION

Depth perception ability is very critical to anticipate the timing of the stroke and the rhythm of the crew. Any compromise in depth perception ability will certainly contribute to decreased performance, as it may affect the anticipation of the relative distances of the fellow competitors.

BINOCULAR VISION

Binocular vision enhances peripheral awareness and provides good depth perception ability. Good binocular vision is more demanding during the end of the race when most attempts are made to reach the target and visual, mental and physical fatigue start affecting performance.

CENTRAL-PERIPHERAL AWARENESS

Central-peripheral awareness is important in racing conditions to maintain awareness of the whereabouts of the other boats and navigational markers. Typically, in rowing peripheral awareness is important to maintain aiming. Therefore, in rowing it is important to know not only how well the rower sees in the periphery of his vision but also how quickly he can react to a peripheral stimulus.

EYE-HAND COORDINATION

Sports like sailing, where repetitive motion is more important than the quick reflexes, can improve sailor's agility, endurance and eye-hand coordination skill. These activities can help develop shoulder's muscles as well as thighs muscle to some degree.

GLARE RECOVERY

The fast glare recovery is not very critical in rowing. But the danger from solar radiation is a known fact, although water is a poor reflector of radiation, but the specular reflection off a sunlit sea can be very intense. The immediate main consideration in competitive sport is not the long-term risk, but the complete physical efficiency during the competition. Visual stress can have a marked effect on physical performance. Besides, if the brain is using all its spare capacity to interpret a degraded ocular image, there will be less energy left to deal with tactics and anticipation. Therefore, glare protection glasses may be useful during the competitions.

Yachting is for everyone, not just for collegiate and Olympic athletes. It is an all-weather activity, which can be enjoyed round the year and by persons of all ages. Those who are not able to express their talent effectively in any other sport, may try yachting as their alternate choice. As far as ocular injuries are concerned, direct impact to the eyes are rare while sailing. More commonly sailors can be knocked in the head or face, sometimes they may be tipped out of the boat. However, the most concerned factor for sailor's eye protection is UV exposure. In addition, water may also be splashed into the eye while sailing but that will cause temporary irritation than injury. Eye protection used for UV exposure will prevent any probable impact as well as water splashing into the eyes.

Visual Demands in Scuba Diving

24 CHAPTER

TERMINOLOGIES

Ascent, Back roll, Bootie, Buddy, Buoyancy, Depth gauge, Fins, Mask

Scuba diving is a sport in which the athlete swims underwater for extended periods using special equipment's. The word "scuba" is actually an acronym for "self-contained underwater breathing apparatus". Scuba diving can also be a very relaxing sport. One learns to dive more quickly than any other sport. It is also suitable for people with physical disability as long as they can propel themselves under the water. Light rays are scattered and absorbed under the water. The light absorption increases as you go deeper into the water. The selective absorption of light wavelengths occurs at varying depths, causing change in color perception. Red color or longer wavelength disappear first at about 30 feet, yellow at 75 feet, and only blue and green remain at depths below 100 feet. There is a change that occur with refraction of light by the eye under water. Water has a high refractive index than air and is similar to that of the cornea. Light entering the cornea from the water hardly refracts, leaving the eye's crystalline lens to focus the light. This leads to very severe hypermetropia. People with severe myopia, therefore, can see better under the water without mask than a normal sighted people. Diving mask or diving helmets solve this problem by enacting an air space in front of the diver's eyes. The refractive error created by the water is mostly corrected by the light travels from water to air through a flat lens, except that the object appears bigger and closer than they actually are, resulting in reduction in field of view.

The importance of various elements of visual system in Scuba Diving can be understood by following description:

VISUAL ACUITY

Dynamic visual acuity is important for tracking the marine life you are observing, the prey you may be hunting and for viewing underwater landscape as you swim through it **(Fig. 24.1)**. Static visual acuity is also equally important to fixate and study an object of interest. Scattering of the light energy by particles suspended in the water and the absorption of different wavelengths cause blurring of the outline of the objects, and thereby reducing the contrast. Color perception is affected due to selective absorption of wavelengths and the clarity of the water.

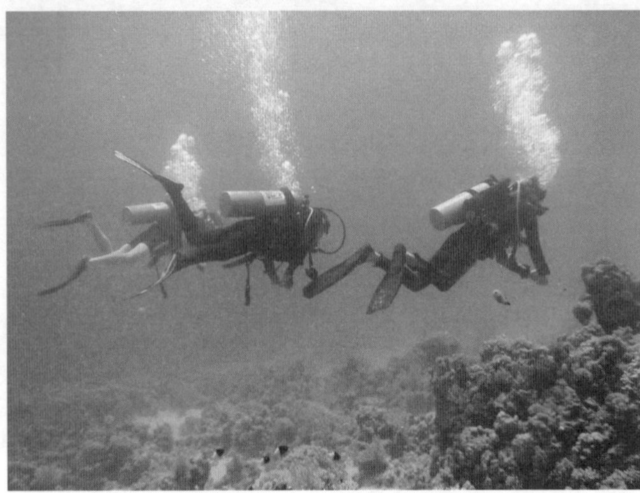

Fig. 24.1: Dynamic visual acuity is important for tracking the marine life.

ACCOMMODATION–VERGENCE FUNCTION

Focus flexibility is important during diving as the divers always need to change his focus to ensure safety and effective hunting under the water.

OCULOMOTOR SKILL

It is one of the key skills used during underwater hunting. Saccades and pursuits both are important. Fixation on the target is also very critical for studying any object under the water which is affected because of poor contrast.

DEPTH PERCEPTION

Overall depth perception is important to the divers when wanting to grasp, touch, or pick up something, and is obviously affected by the increase in magnification of images underwater **(Fig. 24.2)**.

BINOCULAR VISION

Good binocular vision is important as it provides depth perception ability and enhances visual acuity.

CENTRAL-PERIPHERAL AWARENESS

Central-peripheral awareness is the most important visual function in scuba diving, particularly for safety aspect to be aware of dangerous marine life and oncoming boats. If you close your eyes, it may be easy to lose the sense of orientation because you are floating freely in the water and proprioceptive cues are minimum. Peripheral awareness is also an important aiming cue. However, this is often compromised due to face mask.

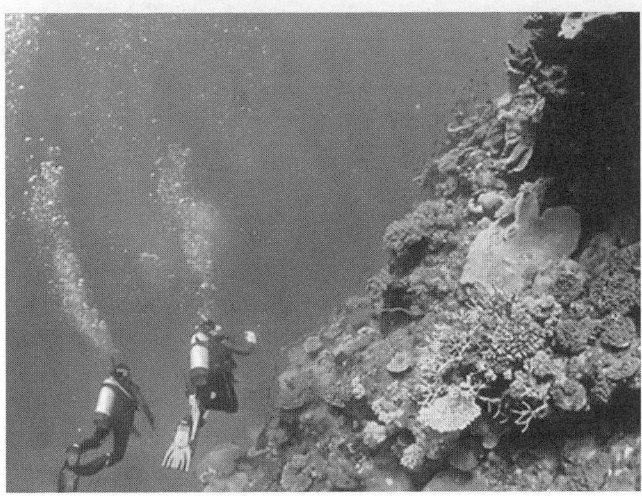

Fig. 24.2: Depth perception is important to grasp, touch or pick things.

EYE-HAND-BODY COORDINATION

This is important to maintain the desired position in the underwater environment.

GLARE RECOVERY

There is minimal glare underwater, making it a less significant factor in scuba diving.

During scuba diving exposure to ambient pressures greater than sea level may result in various disorders and complications, some of them may have ocular manifestations. Diving is hazardous for patients who have undergone ocular surgery. There is a theoretical possibility for corneal rupture in divers following surgery, however, the pressure differential required to produce this effect is extremely high.

Visual Demands in Swimming

25 CHAPTER

TERMINOLOGIES

Freestyle, Dolphin kick, Tumble turn, Somersaults, Body roll, Glide, Lane, Backstroke

Swimming is arguably the only sport that provides opportunities for people of all ages and abilities to participate, at all levels, whether it is recreational, acquiring a life skill, to maintain health and fitness, enjoying water-based activities safely, achieving personal goals or winning medals on the world stage. It can be indoors as well as outdoors. It can be played in chlorinated pools or fresh water or ocean beaches or lakes.

The athlete moves the arms and legs to push against the water and propel himself forward. This is called *swimming strokes*. These strokes may of different types like Butterfly, breaststroke, crawl, sidestroke, backstroke, etc.

BREASTSTROKE

Breaststroke is one of the most restful stroke, done in combination with the breaststroke kick. When the breaststroke is performed correctly, your head comes well above the water and there is plenty of time to take a breath **(Fig. 25.1)**.

BACKSTROKE

Backstroke is another restful stroke as your face is always out of the water and breathing is easy **(Fig. 25.2)**. It is like lying on your back with legs outstretched

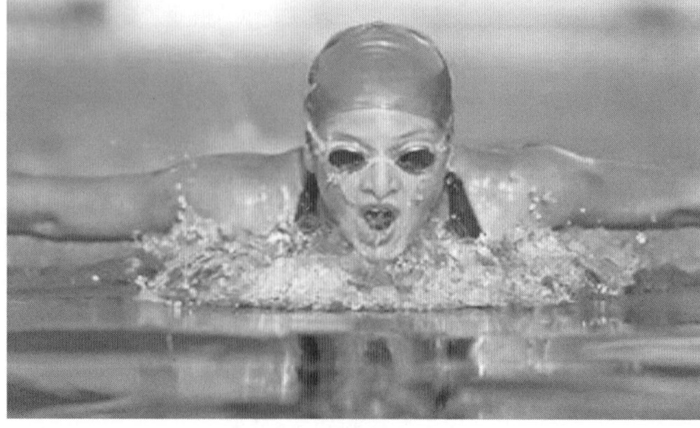

Fig. 25.1: Breaststroke.

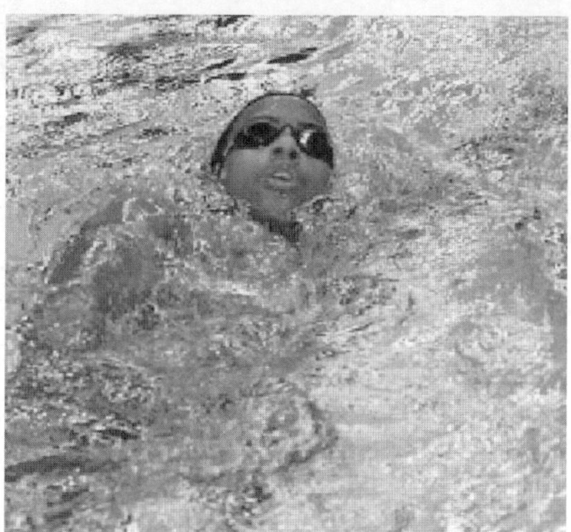

Fig. 25.2: Backstroke.

and head pillowed on water. The arms move in a windmill fashion, while one arm propels the other recover and the legs do the flutter kick.

FRONT CRAWL

This is the fastest and the most popular stroke of all. The arms move in a circular motion in combination with the flutter kick. While one arm propels, the other recovers **(Fig. 25.3)**.

BUTTERFLY STROKE

This is the most difficult stroke. Greater physical strength is required, which renders the stroke unsuitable for long distance. In this stroke, both arms work together, simultaneously and symmetrically and legs operate together to make two dolphin kicks during each arm cycle.

SIDESTROKE

The sidestroke is done on your side with one ear in the water, the head rests on your arm which is extended out ahead of you, with palm facing downwards. The other arm is kept on your side.

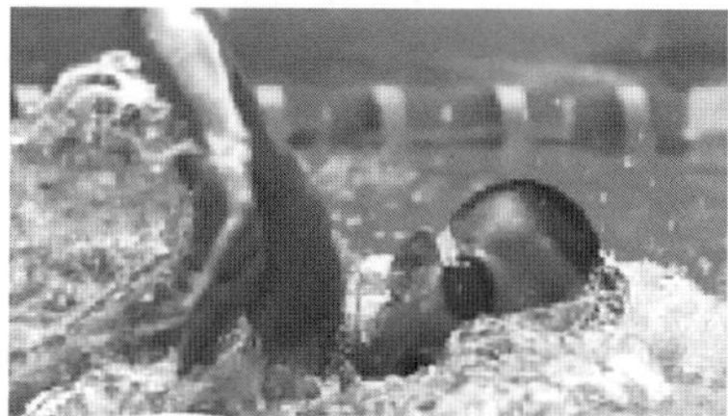

Fig. 25.3: Front crawl.

With all the strokes except the backstroke, the eyes mostly remain under water. Hence vision is not so critical in swimming, except in backstroke. Whatever the visual need is thought in swimming that suggests anticipation is predominant. The swimmer needs to be able to adjust to anticipate very accurately, the distance from the turn and in backstroke, to judge their position in relation to the ceiling joists. It is also important to be able to see other competitors before and during the race. In most of the strokes the swimmer must keep his head above the surface of the water except underwater swimming. The only time he swims under the water is the first stroke after the start and each turn. Backstroke swimming involves alternate over the head arm strokes and flutter kick in a supine position. The use of eyes in backstroke swimming is very important to swim in a straight line. If the swimmer is swimming in indoor pool, it may be easier to sight on something overhead, like a railing or the line where the walls and the ceiling meet each other. On the other hand, if you are swimming backstroke in an outdoor pool, it gets a little tougher to swim in straight line. Although it is hard to avoid, but try and not to sight on clouds, birds or jet planes flying over the pool. Instead, look for something that runs parallel to the direction you are swimming. It could be a power line or a telephone line, the top of a fence or wall or a row of bleachers. At lower eye levels, possibly right at the water level, you will need to use your peripheral vision to see the opponent's position.

The importance of various elements of visual system in Swimming can be understood by following description:

■ VISUAL ACUITY

Visual acuity is useful for orientation and mobility before and after a race. It may also play some role in judging distances and determining the time of the turn, although the level of visual acuity needed under water has not yet been established.

■ ACCOMMODATION–VERGENCE FUNCTION

As far as swimming is concerned accommodation and vergence function is least important.

■ OCULOMOTOR SKILL

Fixation may be considered to be important only while entry into the water. Besides, during backstroke vestibular and pursuit eye movement may be considered to know the position of the fellow competitors.

■ DEPTH PERCEPTION

Depth perception may be useful to anticipate the distance of turns and curbs and judging the distance while jumping into the water during the start.

BINOCULAR VISION

The presence of binocular vision may be thought to provide good peripheral awareness on both sides of the swimmer.

CENTRAL-PERIPHERAL AWARENESS

Central-peripheral awareness is an important skill in competitive swimming for self-direction within the lane and for continually processing the status of the rest of the competitors. This is also essential to align during whatever aiming is needed in swimming.

EYE-HAND COORDINATION

Some eye-hand coordination is needed in backstroke, breaststroke and butterfly where hand must touch the wall during turn.

GLARE RECOVERY

Swimmers usually wear swimming goggles, hence glare has no role in swimming.

Swimming is a difficult area of sport, because of the classical concern of *Acanthamoeba*. Protection from chemical conjunctivitis and waterborne microbes is very important. Those swimmers who require vision correction ideally should use contact lenses with plano swim goggle over it. Some swimmers are more comfortable with prescription swimming goggle rather than contact lenses. Keeping the chlorine water off their cornea while underwater provides clearer vision and a better safety profile. Every swimmer knows that the water gets in at some point during the training session and generally they do not take their contact lenses out to have a shower afterwards, so this is another area where best clinical practice needs to be tempered with common sense.

Visual Demands in Rifle Shooting

26 CHAPTER

TERMINOLOGIES

Bullets, Cartridge, Shot, Trigger

Rifle shooting is a target sport that requires good physical and psychological conditioning. It can be played indoors as well as outdoors. At elite level, rifle shooting requires many years of practice and training to reach the exceptionally high standard required for competition shooting. Although physical endurance and stamina are also important, it is more of a mind game than of a physical. There are some fundamental rules that the shooter must practice and these rules are given below:

- Relax
- Feel the presence of target
- Breathe normally
- Control movement
- Clear his mind
- Control trigger and
- Follow through

In rifle shooting, the participants fire from either a prone, a standing or a kneeling position, earning points with his shots at 10 ring target for the center ring, 9 for the next one, and so on **(Fig. 26.1)**. The score in the final round is added to the competitor's score in the qualification round and the winner is the competitor with the most points at the end of the match.

There are 5 contact points between the rifle and the body:

1. The first point of contact is at the butt plate and the shoulder joint. It is important that it does not slip off.
2. The right hand and the grip would be the second contact point. It must be firm.
3. The left arm should make contact with the gun as it is lifted up. As the left elbow falls into place on the hip, take note of the balance and weight distribution on the feet.
4. The fourth contact point is between the cheek and the cheekpiece. The above four points must be checked before the fifth contact point is established.
5. The fifth contact point is between the trigger finger and the trigger blade. Premature placement of the finger on the trigger might cause an accidental firing of the gun so one must always remember to do this last.

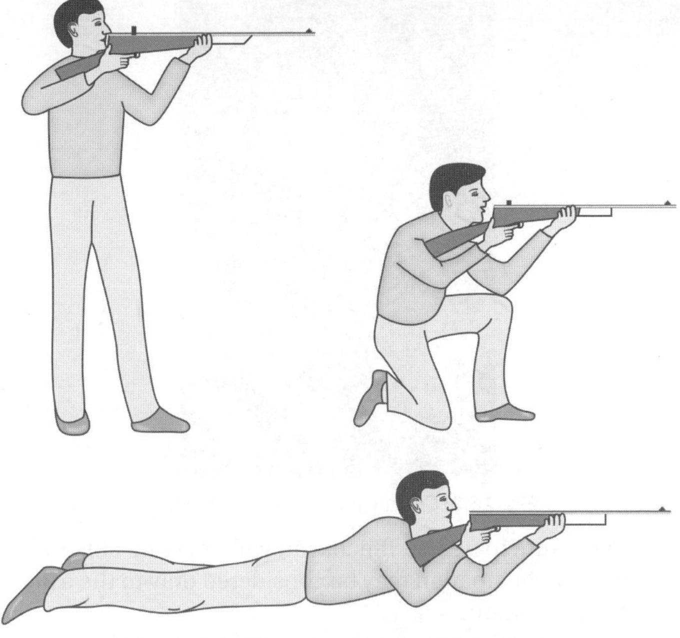

Fig. 26.1: Different position in rifle shooting.

The main event in rifle shooting is repetitive in nature and is spread over a period of time. In this respect, it is a non-dynamic sport. It is a highly visually dependent sport with a particular importance to eye dominance. Good vision is very important in lining up the gun's sight with the target. Predominantly it is an aiming sport. The shooter has to align the front sight and the rear sight perfectly and consistently. There are four things in this equation and these are:

1. Aiming eye
2. The rear sight
3. The front sight, and
4. The target.

The athlete peeps through the sights, and sees three circles. He has to align these circles concentrically with the target in the middle. Don't expect the gun to stop moving completely. The goal is to minimize its movement. The ideal motion of the gun is circular. The sights will just play around the target. Unlike pistol, it is very important to have a clear picture of the sights than the target in rifle shooting. Once the sights have stabilized, pressure must be applied to the trigger to release the shot. After the shot has been released, the shooter must maintain the sight picture for a few seconds. This follow through is needed to be able to see what possible errors occurred during the release of the shot.

The target in rifle shooting is stationary at a predecided distance. The shooter takes time to align the sights with the target before the shot is being released. It is, therefore, an aiming sport **(Fig. 26.2)**. Anticipation is not very

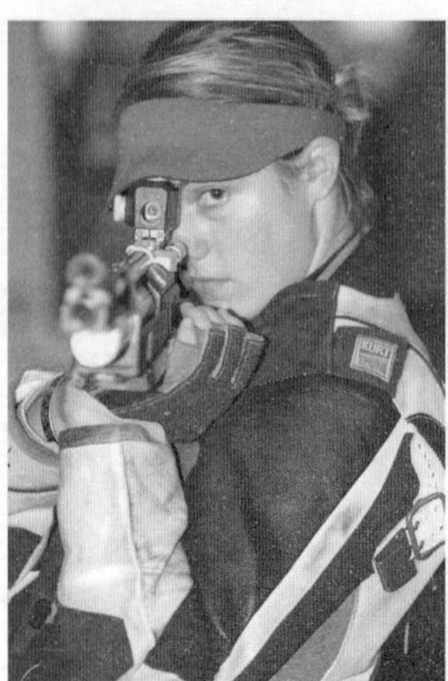

Fig. 26.2: Critical aiming in rifle shooting.

important. If you anticipate and flinch, you will never be able to shoot well. The importance of anticipation may be considered only to the extent needed for eye-hand coordination.

The importance of various elements of visual system in Rifle Shooting can be understood by following description:

VISUAL ACUITY (FIG. 26.3)

The rifle shooter must place the rear peep sight, the front sight aperture and the target in line before shooting. In order to align correctly, it is most important to have a good focus on the front sight aperture. The target should also be clear but never at the expense of the front sight. The rear sight serves as a pinhole aperture for the system, so it may not be in focus. Very fine acuity

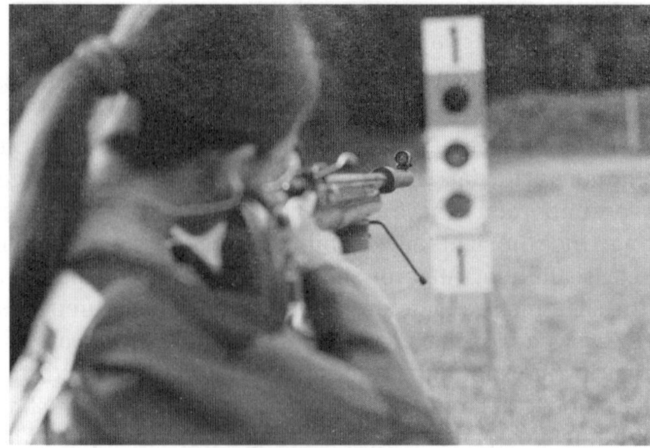

Fig. 26.3: Rifle shooter must place the rear peep sight, the front sight aperture and the target in line before shooting.

is needed to align the sighting pattern. Static visual acuity is more important than dynamic visual acuity. The use of hyperacuity, i.e., vernier acuity while aligning the system enhances the performance. Contrast may be an issue, depending on the lighting over the shooters head. Shooters may have different sized rear aperture sights to change the amount of light getting through to the shooters eye. In fact, some rifle shooters may wear an adjustable mechanical iris or an occluder attachment on their glasses to control the light getting into the eye. Color vision is not very critical.

ACCOMMODATION–VERGENCE FUNCTION

In rifle shooting, the target distance is fixed and the distance between the sights does not change. Only possibility is that the distance between the eye to rear sight may change which must be avoided. So accommodation–vergence facility is not very critical.

OCULOMOTOR SKILL

Shooting may take long periods of visual concentration on the target which is done with just one eye which establishes the importance of fixation ability on the target.

DEPTH PERCEPTION

The target in rifle shooting is stationary at a predefined distance, allowing for precious time to align the sights with the target and the shot to be taken. Also the shooter usually covers his non dominant eye with some sort of occluder to prevent any distraction from that eye. Therefore, depth perception may not be very critical for a rifle shooter.

BINOCULAR VISION

The attributes of good binocular vision are better visual acuity and high contrast which are very important for rifle shooting. In this respect it may be considered an important visual element. Usually shooter closes their non-dominant eye to aim at the target. But closing one eye to aim at the target deprives them from the many advantages of binocular vision **(Fig. 26.4)**. Long periods of visual concentration on the target results in high amount of eye strain which may not occur when the aiming is done with both eyes open. To prevent any distraction from non-dominant eye, the shooter may place some sort of blinder over that eye. The ideal blinder blocks out any vision of the non-aiming eye but still lets light through to that eye. It is important for light to get to the non-aiming eye to keep the eyes from dilating which may cut down on the depth of focus of the shooter.

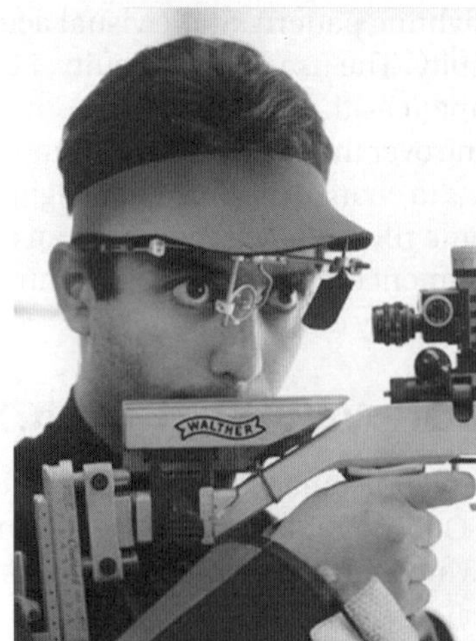

Fig. 26.4: Aiming with two eyes open.

CENTRAL-PERIPHERAL AWARENESS

Good central vision is very essential for a rifle shooter. Peripheral awareness is not very critical. A very small field of view is required for target shooting. In fact, side shields are placed on the sides of the glasses or a hat to blockout any peripheral movement and help the shooter concentrate on the task of aligning the target bulls-eye with the pinhole-like sights. Only time when the shooter is using his peripheral vision is while aligning the front sight in the center of the rear sight aperture.

EYE-HAND-BODY COORDINATION

In rifle shooting, rifle is in contact with the body from 5 points, which makes eye-hand-body coordination a very important skill, although not purely visual. This is a sport which puts extreme emphasis on eye-hand-body coordination. The fine motor control needed for aiming and shot release have to be perfected to an almost unimaginable degree to hit the target to score maximum points.

GLARE RECOVERY

There is not much concern for the glare and any other radiation exposure, as in today's competitive level, if the rifle match is played outdoors, the shooter shoots from under a covered shelter and also uses protective caps and glasses that protects them from these elements.

Shooting, in general requires a high visual demand which is much beyond the imagination of a general person. The shooter is in furious dynamic equilibrium with all muscles in constantly readjusting mode. Visual fatigue has a profound effect on the ability to see the object of interest clearly. If visual perception is not reliable, then the resulting delay in releasing the shot adds to physical and mental fatigue. But interesting aspect of shooting apart from predominantly an aiming sport, especially rifle and pistol is that the target may not be necessarily clear. The technique rifle and pistol shooter mostly use, is to focus on the foresight of the gun or the rifle, and align this centrally in the blur of the target. As long as the blurred target is uniformly round, its edges do not have to be defined. As far as safety is concerned when shooting a rifle there is always the risk of defective ammunition backfiring and propelling debris back at the shooter. It is necessary for the shooter to wear eye protection to stop this debris from entering the eye. If at all possible side shields should be used to further protect the shooter from debris.

Visual Demands in Clay Pigeon Shooting

27 CHAPTER

TERMINOLOGIES

Clay target, Lead, Range, Shotgun, Trap, Launch

Clay pigeon is a shooting sport where in flying targets are shot with a shotgun **(Fig. 27.1)**. The sport is termed clay pigeon as it used to be played by hitting live pigeon in the past. Now, the live pigeons have been replaced by similar looking flying targets projected by designated machines. The targets are usually made of clay in black or white or any fluorescent color and are easily broken by the hit. There are three main forms of clay pigeon shooting:

1. **Trap shooting**: Targets are thrown either as singles or doubles from one or more traps situated nearly 15 m in front of the shooter and are generally going away from the firing point at varying speeds, angles and elevations.
2. **Skeet shooting**: Targets are thrown in singles and doubles from 2 trap houses situated nearly 40 meters apart, at opposite ends of a semicircular arc on which there are seven shooting positions. The targets are thrown at set trajectories and speeds.
3. **Clay shooting**: Targets are thrown in a great variety of trajectories, angles, speeds, elevations and distances.

The athlete lines up and stands at designated firing marks, facing the trap and taking the stance by placing the feet in relation to the area where he plans to shoot the target. Perfect stance is very important to enable smooth and free movement and to ensure smooth follow through with movement of gun. The gun at the point of firing must be at the shoulder of the shooter. The shooter then looks for the target and shoots it to break the target into fragments. Three

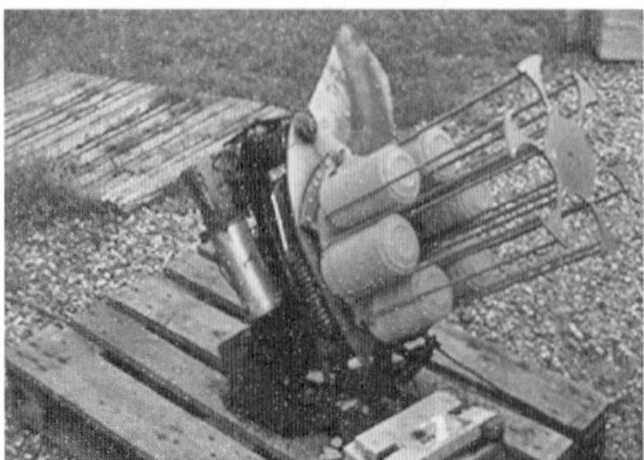

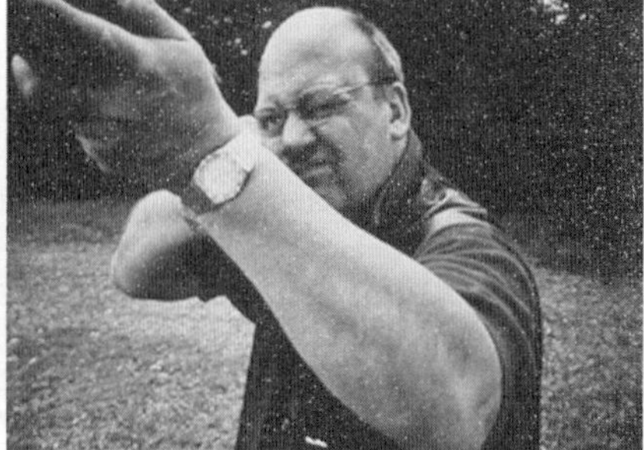

Fig. 27.1: Clay shooting.

points are awarded for a single barrel kill, two points for second barrel kill and zero for the loss; 25 lays are shot, allowing a maximum score of 75 points.

Clay pigeon shooting is a controlled sport. The sporting task is same for all the participants and is repetitive. During the extended competition, the consistency of performance is more important than hitting the target once. As the day passes, the effect of visual fatigue like eye strain, epiphora, tension, headache, retinal bleaching may begin to accumulate, their aiming is most likely to be affected.

Clay pigeon is primarily an anticipatory sport, the shooter anticipates the direction and the speed of the clay through the air and then brings his gun to aim at the target to break it. To achieve the perfect aiming, the shooter stands at the designated firing marks, facing the trap and adopts shooting stance, puts his feet in relation to the area where he plans to shoot the target. Alignment of the feet and body with the peripheral awareness of the trap house gives a clue for aiming.

The importance of various elements of visual system in Clay Pigeon Shooting can be understood by following description:

VISUAL ACUITY

Both static and dynamic visual acuity are important in clay pigeon because of the importance of aiming in an anticipatory dominant sport. The target size is small and are thrown from the traps at very high speed, which necessitates the need of high contrast. Usually, the colors of the target are predefined, therefore, color perception is not very important. Wind speed and its direction may also have some influence on the visual acuity.

ACCOMMODATION–VERGENCE FUNCTION

The shooter needs to be able to focus on the moving clay and accuracy of the focusing ability may be affected by tiredness especially if there is a problem using the two eyes together. Daylong event requires huge amount of sustained accommodation facility. Fast focusing on target is very critical in clay shooting.

OCULOMOTOR SKILL

In clay shooting, the eyes need to be able to focus on a moving clay. Fixation ability together with pursuit, saccade and vestibular movements are important for the shooter. The clays are released from the trap at a speed which makes saccades the most critical among all the oculomotor skills.

DEPTH PERCEPTION

Depth perception is important to anticipate the speed, direction and distance of the target. In clay shooting, the target is moving and the shooter is aware of the barrel more than the target. He calls for the target which has to be shot in a fraction of second through the air. Accurate, fast and intelligent depth perception is probably most important skill to aim correctly especially in clay shooting.

BINOCULAR VISION

Binocular vision is important to anticipate the speed and the direction of the target through the air. Good binocular vision also improves contrast and peripheral awareness which are important skills in clay shooting. Even the correction in amblyopic eye is critical which have a critical input in the ability to judge depth.

CENTRAL-PERIPHERAL AWARENESS

Central-peripheral awareness is very critical in clay pigeon as it facilitates both anticipation and aiming. The barrel of the gun which facilitates aiming at the target is no doubt at the center of their vision, but they will never be seen when the trigger is shot. But keeping the barrel in sight is very important to aim correctly in moving target sport. Peripheral awareness is the skill which facilitates it. The importance of the skill can be understood with the fact that even if the target is shot or missed, the barrel-target relationship has to be maintained.

EYE-HAND-BODY COORDINATION

Clay pigeon events take place while standing and the body moves to follow the moving clay. The clay is being fired from the trap on the call of the shooter who is ready with the rifle positioned in the shoulder. The body is perfectly positioned on the firing line with feet firmly placed. The visual input from the eyes has to be translated into spatial location by the brain which informs the various muscles of the body to move in such a way as to enable the shooter to aim accurately and fire precisely.

GLARE RECOVERY

The expert clay shooter, apart from requiring steady hands, strength and concentration, will need to have excellent eye sight to be able to recover fast from the glare. The glare may disrupt the aiming and result in poor performance. In clay shooting, the shooters usually use filter glasses to protect their eyes from the fragments of clay. These glasses have glare protection properties also.

Clay pigeon is a visually demanding sport where primary vision accounts for 10% of the visual task, whereas peripheral vision accounts for rest 90%. Shouldering a gun becomes a habit through practice, it is not too difficult in the early stages to change shoulder, to maintain natural eye dominance. So far as safety is concerned clay shooter always play the sport with protective eyewear. There is always a possibility of eye injury because of the fragments of the clay.

Visual Demands in Archery

28 CHAPTER

TERMINOLOGIES

Bow, Arrow, Draw, Field Archery, Gold, Nock, Sling

Archery is a game of bow and arrow. It is played by men and women both. The archer needs to shoot the arrow at the designated target at different distances. He gets 6 shots for each distance. The target in general consists of 10 circles with the center one known as Gold. Top class archer concentrates to aim at the Gold, to score 10 points. Thus, the main action is repetitive in nature and is spread over a long day. Hitting correctly at Gold once is not the ultimate skill of a top archer. It is the consistency over the days long game which differentiates a great archer from a good archer. In this respect archery is a controlled sport.

The archer stands upright with one foot each side of the shooting line, takes an arrow and put it onto the bowstring, holds the bow with one hand and draws the string with another, keeping the elbow of the drawing arm as high as possible and the index finger touching to the center of the chin. He closes the non-dominant eye and peeps through the peep sight with the dominant eye to the tip of the arrow at bow and sights at the target. That's how the archer achieves aiming. Anticipation helps to judge the distance of the target and to decide the extent to which the string is to be drawn. So, archery is predominantly an aiming sport where anticipation is important to prevent undershoot **(Fig. 28.1)**.

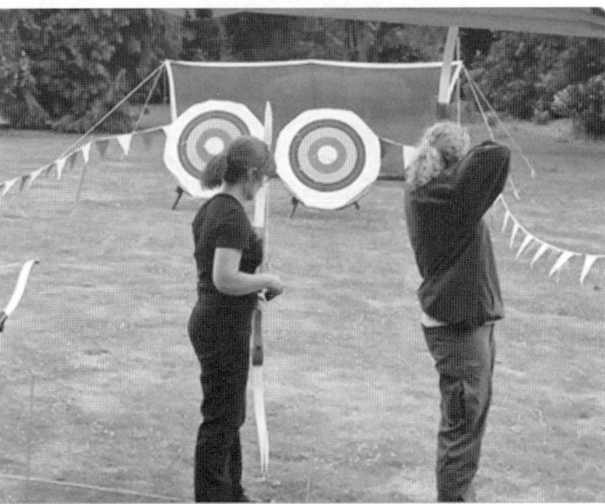

Fig. 28.1: Aiming and anticipation in archery.

The importance of various elements of visual system in Archery can be understood by following description:

VISUAL ACUITY

Archery involves shooting arrows at a fixed target set at a fixed distance **(Fig. 28.2)**. So, static visual acuity is more important than dynamic visual acuity. The good visual acuity will provide crisp and clear vision to aim at the distant target. If vision is compromised, then aiming will be disrupted resulting in poor performance. Besides, the long-sustained clear vision is more important to have a consistent performance. Demand of good vision necessitates good contrast, the need of which increases as the day passes. Color perception is not very important.

ACCOMMODATION-VERGENCE FUNCTION

Accommodation-vergence facility is not an important skill in archery. However, the only time the skill becomes important when the archer looks through the peep sight and then to the target.

OCULOMOTOR SKILL

Fixation at the target is very important skill in archery. Eye movements are not very important skills in archery.

DEPTH PERCEPTION

Depth perception is an important visual skill as it affects anticipation which is very important skill to prevent over and under estimation of target distance.

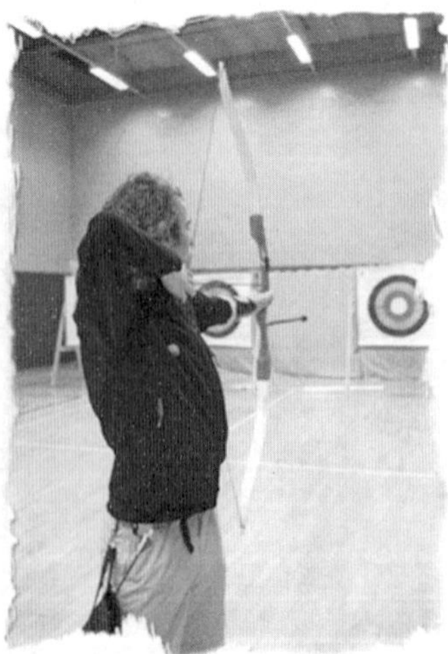

Fig. 28.2: Fixed target at a fixed distance.

BINOCULAR VISION

Binocular vision is important as it gives better vision than monocular vision and improves contrast and also facilitates depth perception.

CENTRAL-PERIPHERAL AWARENESS

Central vision is more important for fixation at the target. Peripheral awareness is not very critical.

EYE-HAND-FOOT-BODY COORDINATION

Archer should place their feet comfortably and firmly apart and point them at right angle to the target. A right-handed archer holds the bow grip with the left hand. The archer fits the arrow into the bowstring, rests it on the left side of the bow, and raises the bow to a vertical position. The bowstring is usually drawn back with the middle three fingers of the right hand, keeping the arrow between the first and second fingers. At full draw, the string touches the archer's chin. The archer, then releases the arrow and remains still until the arrow hits the target. The entire sequence of procedure from holding of bow to releasing of arrow and the follow through necessitates steady eye-hand-body coordination **(Fig. 28.3)**. It seems deceptively an easy sport where aiming at the target is needed but actually this is not true. Hand-eye coordination, body control, trained muscles, drawing and aiming of the arrow, hand relaxation, arm strength and steadiness are required for successful target hitting. A good stance is essential to distribute the weight of the body which is essential for consistent performance.

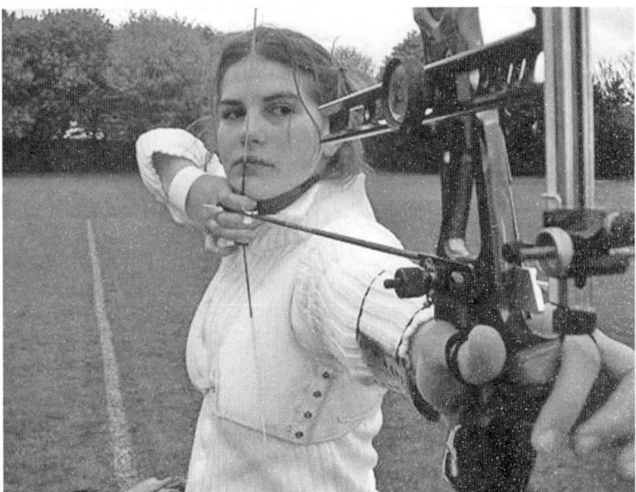

Fig. 28.3: Hand-eye coordination and body control is required for drawing and aiming of the arrow.

GLARE RECOVERY

Archery is an aiming sport, usually played outdoor on day long format. The archer is exposed to the bright sunlight which can cause glare. The archer might use glare protection glasses during the event to prevent eyes from glare.

Vision appears to affect archer's performance in most fundamental way. Visual fatigue, mental and physical are likely to have effect on the sporting skill. Archery is usually a safe game; ocular injuries have not been reported.

Visual Demands in Chess

29 CHAPTER

TERMINOLOGIES

Check, Checkmate, Chessboard, Fork, Bishop, King, Pawn, Rook, Castle, Gambit

Chess is a recreational and competitive sport for two players **(Fig. 29.1)**. It is played on a square chequered chessboard with 64 squares. It is played in an indoor environment. At the start, each player controls 16 pieces—one king, one queen, two rooks, two knights, two bishops and eight pawns. The objective of the game is to checkmate the opponent's king. The game does not have to necessarily end in checkmate. The player may resign if the situation looks hopeless or it may end in draw by agreement. Chess is advocated as a way of enhancing mental prowess. It has long been associated with strategic thinking and problem solving. Chess enthusiasts have long argued that playing the chess leads to improved scholastic attainment and greater self-confidence. It is also argued that playing chess develops the skill of creative and critical thinking and the ability to concentrate and solve problems. Chess, by its features, is a controlled sport. But it is no way less competitive than any other explosive sport for the huge demand of mental extremes including intense concentration, furrowed brow, tightened diaphragm, multi-level inward thinking, sequential processing, stress and autonomic response involved in the sport. The player's body is held in a controlled position while the eyes co-ordinate precisely at places on the chessboard and the mind is feeding back a complicated image of spatial awareness and position. It all appears

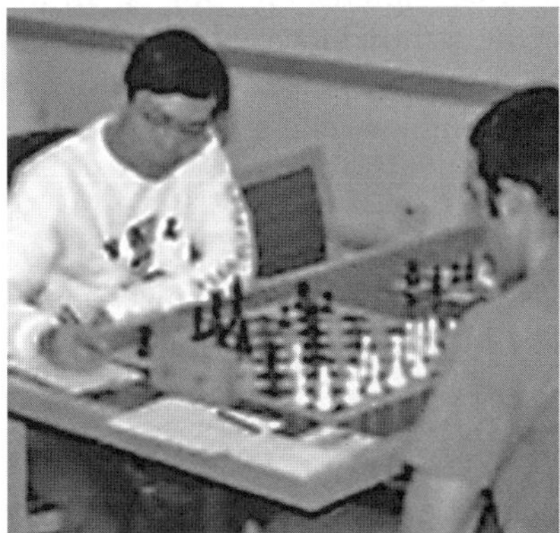

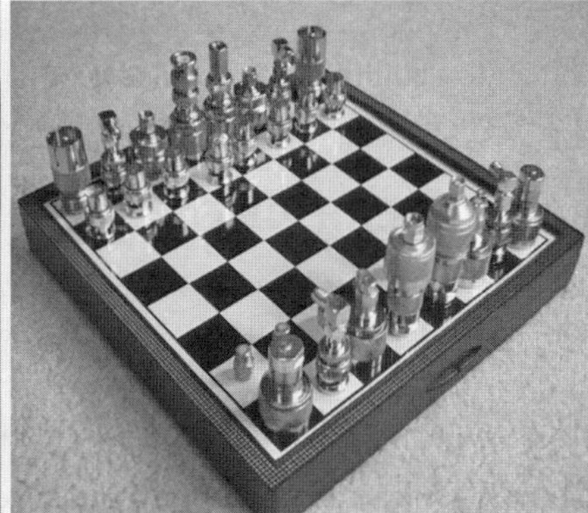

Fig. 29.1: Game of chess.

to be static but is in fact in dynamic equilibrium. Chess is predominantly an anticipating sport. However, anticipation in this sport is predominantly linked to the anticipation of the next move of the opponent. A player may visualize the next move and its impact ahead of time so that he can plan his attack or defense accordingly. Although anticipation is more important than aiming, visual aiming and anticipation—both seem to be relatively less important factor in chess as compare to other sports.

The importance of various elements of visual system in Chess can be understood by following description:

VISUAL ACUITY

Static visual acuity is more important than dynamic visual acuity to see the positions of pieces on the chess board. Color perception may not be very important because of the predecided set of colors used for the game. High contrast will add to the visual clarity. Visual acuity may be affected by indoor light level, position of the luminaries, reflectivity of the chessboard surface.

ACCOMMODATION-VERGENCE FUNCTION

Focus flexibility is not very critical in chess, but because of the intense concentration, the players have tendency to be esophoric.

OCULOMOTOR SKILL

In chess there is a little ocular movement and a lot of concentration is needed which makes fixation ability a very critical factor. Other than fixation saccades are used to observe the positions of pieces on the chessboard.

DEPTH PERCEPTION

There is definitely an element of spatial reasoning to chess or other similar game, but it has nothing to do with depth perception ability of the visual system which is critical to manipulate three-dimensional objects in the mind. The black and white squares make the game a lot easier for the depth perception ability. One can easily count the squares and figureout the moves. Depth perception is not related to spatial reasoning in chess.

BINOCULAR VISION

It is always better to have good binocular vision because this maximizes acuity, contrast sensitivity, and stops the muscles around the eyes from getting tired.

CENTRAL-PERIPHERAL AWARENESS

Central vision is more important as the player always keeps his focus right on to the chessboard. The players would always like to overlook what is happening in their periphery so that they can concentrate more on the chess board and the next move of the opponent.

■ EYE-HAND-BODY COORDINATION

The player's body is held in a controlled position while the eyes co-ordinate precisely at places on the chessboard and the mind is feeding back a complicated image of spatial awareness and position. It all appears to be static but is in fact in dynamic equilibrium.

■ GLARE RECOVERY

The chess player gets enough time to play his next move, hence glare recovery is not very important in chess.

It is widely acknowledged that chess is the best example of an intellectual activity among the games. Although practice had the influence on the chess skill, intelligence explains some variance even after the inclusion of practice. The outcome of the match totally depends on the player's intelligence and imagining power. Luck does not play any role and if a player loses, he can only blame himself, or his intelligence, not being smart enough to understand opponent's move.

Visual Demands in Snooker

30 CHAPTER

TERMINOLOGIES

Frames, Cue, Baize, Baulk line, Bridge, Miscue, Pocket

Snooker is a cue sport that is played on a large baize-covered table with pockets in each of the four corners and in the middle of each of the long side cushions. A regulation table of 12 feet × 6 feet is used. It is played using a cue, one white ball (the cue ball), 15 red balls (worth 1 point each) and 6 balls of different colors (worth 2-7 points each). A player wins a frame of snooker by scoring more points than the opponent, using cue ball to pot the red and colored balls. A match consists of a previously agreed number of frames.

At the start of a frame the balls are positioned and the players take it in turns to hit a shot, their aim being to pot one of the red balls and score a point. If they do pot a red ball, that red ball remains in the pocket and they are allowed another shot, this time the aim being to pot one of the colored balls. If successful, they must try to pot another red ball. This process continues until they fail to pot the desired ball, at which point their opponent comes back to the table to play the next shot. The game continues in this manner until all reds are potted and only 6 colorballs are left on the table. Finally, all the colored balls are potted and the frame is over. The player with maximum points wins. Thus, the main action of the game is repetitive and spread over a span of time. It is, therefore, a controlled sport, requires lots of patience.

Snooker is highly visually dependent sport requiring almost equal levels of aiming and depth perception and with a particular consideration of eye dominance **(Fig. 30.1)**. When viewing the entire playing surface, the player generally steps back from the table to assess their next shot. Once they address their shot at the table, the visual need is similar to sighting down a rifle barrel. The player focuses at the end of the cue stick, the cue ball and aims the ball at which he is shooting. Then he again anticipates the distance of the ball from the hole where he intends to pot into. In this respect aiming predominates the anticipation, although anticipation is also very important.

The importance of various elements of visual system in Snooker can be understood by following description:

■ VISUAL ACUITY

In snooker, a stationary ball is addressed and propelled towards a stationary target. Static visual acuity is more important than dynamic visual acuity. Any

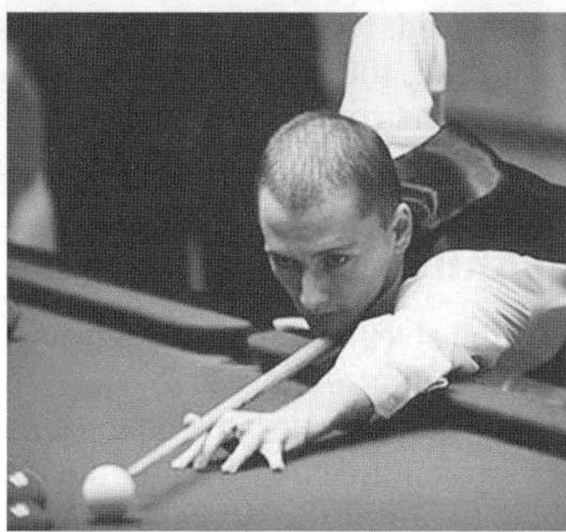

Fig. 30.1: Aiming and anticipating to pot.

uncorrected refractive error may affect the performance as this is highly a visually demanding sport where aiming and anticipation both are important. The game is usually played on a table with green base and red ball, white, blue, black balls. There is a good contrast between the object and their background **(Fig. 30.2)**. Color identification of balls are important to score points in this sport which establishes the implications of color vision in snooker.

ACCOMMODATION–VERGENCE FUNCTION

The predominance of aiming requires good convergence and divergence facility in snooker and the ability to shift focus from near to intermediate distance effectively is particularly linked with potting of the ball. The viewing distance in a snooker game varies within the range of playing surface length, playing surface width and within this viewing distance is mostly confined within the distance from shooting position to end of the cue stick. A player

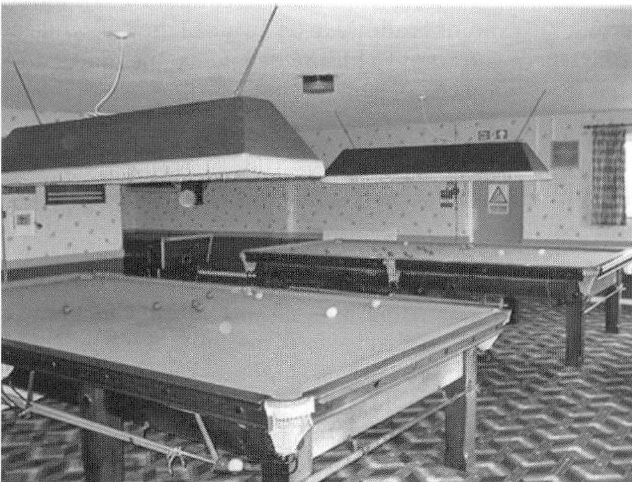

Fig. 30.2: Indoor environment for snooker, needing high contrast.

viewing the ball, therefore, needs to accommodate somewhere between 0.25 D and 1.50 D. During the potting, the player needs to converge constantly onto the cue stick, cue ball and then to object with an eye on the hole, which means long sustained vergence facility is also very critical in snooker.

OCULOMOTOR SKILL

The snooker player must be able to maintain steady fixation while hitting the cue. Any disruption in the fixation ability will severely affect the performance. The ability to focus properly on the cue ball and the target is very essential in making good contact between the cue stick and the cue ball. Fine focusing techniques can help both in hitting the sweet shot and sliding a smoother hit into the pocket.

DEPTH PERCEPTION

Depth perception, probably the most important visual skill in snooker, provides valuable aid in estimating the distance between the object ball and the hole. If the player does not estimate this distance correctly, the player will have a tendency to either hit the ball too short or too hard and possibly too much to the left or right of the hole.

BINOCULAR VISION

Binocular vision is the predisposing factor for the peak performance in snooker. Binocular vision facilitates aiming and depth perception which are very critical in snooker. It also provides better vision and reduces ocular fatigue in a day long match.

CENTRAL-PERIPHERAL AWARENESS

Central-peripheral awareness allows to be aware of the ball while at the same time knowing where you want to hit the ball. Once the player addresses his next shot, it is the central vision which is more critical to aim the ball into the hole.

EYE-HAND-BODY COORDINATION

The player while playing snooker usually stands with his left foot slightly advanced, his left arm extended and resting on the table to form a bridge, and his body, not facing the table squarely, but forming an acute angle with the sides at which he stands. All muscles of his limbs into their usual and most natural posture—as rigidity of body is at all times awkward and ungraceful, and seriously interferes with play. The cue, though allowed to rest loosely in the hand at the time of drawing back, should be held firmly at the moment of contact with the ball; and in all strokes, except the “jump” and “perpendicular force”, the direction of the cue should be maintained as much as possible in the horizontal. The striking motion should be confined to the arm, and chiefly to the lower division of it. All these require huge amount of eye-hand-body coordination. Rock-like stability of the body, firm fixation of the eyes with trombone like arm swinging are the grand essentials of success in snooker.

GLARE RECOVERY

There is no need for UV, infrared, laser or any other form of radiation protection since the game of pool is experienced indoors. Almost all pool table have a low hanging light over the top of it. The lighting can have detrimental effects on the spectacle wearer due to the glare produced. To reduce this glare and possible ghosting effect, it is suggested that the spectacle wearer should have anti-reflection coating on both surface.

Snooker is a slow moving sport and involves each participant taking shots in turns. Surprisingly visual dynamics of snooker are very essential elements for big success. So far safety is concerned ocular injuries are not very common. There is no need for impact protection, side shields, or a specialty lens thickness for the game of pool. To protect the integrity of the ocular surface and tear film, it is advisable not to wear contact lens while playing in areas with heavy smoke in the air, like bar, pool halls, etc. The smoke can dryout contact lenses very quickly, which can lead to eye dryness and discomfort.

Visual Demands in Motor Car Racing

31 CHAPTER

TERMINOLOGIES

Aerodynamics, Airbox, Cockpit, Late braking, Early braking, Marbles, Steering wheel

Motor car is now one of the world's most popular sports involving racing automobiles. Among the many type of car racing, Formula One is the most popular sporting event **(Fig. 31.1)**. This is a single seater racing and is one of the top ten watched sporting event in the world. Formula One is one of the most expensive sports in terms of spending. There are other categories of single seater racing. In a motor car racing sport, the driver is in a furious dynamic equilibrium with all muscles in constantly readjusting mode. The key skill is physiological control against all the elements of metabolism that tend to detract from mental fatigue, blood sugar level, dehydration, muscle fatigue and visual fatigue. The sport might lack the explosion of boxing or for that to say of football or rugby. But the amount of microscopic control and endurance needed makes it a dynamic sport.

Vision and driving skill are directly related. Therefore, care must be directed towards the driver's physiological well-being as much as to the mechanics of the vehicle, and vision is the highest expression of physiological well-being. When it comes to the cost effectiveness, many seconds per lap could be gained simply by attending to driver's visual needs and without an extra expenditure on engine development. The fundamentals of car racing must include driver's entire physiology including his visual performance in addition to car design, engine, chassis, drag and tyres. The preliminary visual skill in car racing is

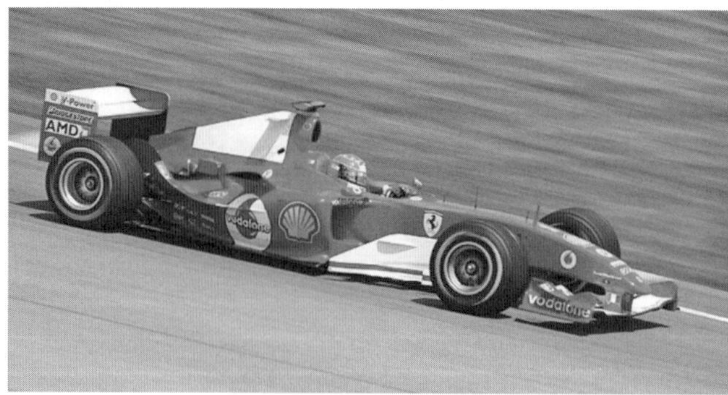

Fig. 31.1: Formula One race.

anticipation by depth perception which facilitates peripheral awareness. The anticipation ability can be further increased if the course is memorized like a musician who can play from memory and does not have to rely on reading notes. Aiming is needed to maintain the position in line. Any disturbance in anticipation may result into turning late on the apex of the turn, missing brake points or a wet patch on the track.

The importance of various elements of visual system in Motor Car Racing can be understood by following description:

VISUAL ACUITY

In a dynamic sport like car racing good level of static visual acuity is desirable. The air in the cockpit is of particular concern since vision is very sensitive to reduced oxygen level in the blood. However, very good acuity might inhibit peripheral awareness, which reacts quickest to visual stimuli. Driving a race car is more visually demanding than everyday driving **(Fig. 31.2)**. If vision breaks down towards the end of the race, it can lead to serious results. A driver must be able to maintain his visual skill level throughout the race. The last few laps of a race are usually the most demanding, when the most attempts at the passing are made. Color perception is important for the drivers to enable them to discern different color flags used by corner workers for communication.

ACCOMMODATION–VERGENCE FUNCTION

Accommodation-vergence is not a very important visual skill for a car racer. A crisp focus for distance as well on the dash is not always essential. However, study has shown that convergence weakness may make things appear further away than they really are and may result in loss of depth perception. This may cause late braking and therefore result in too much speed coming out of the corner.

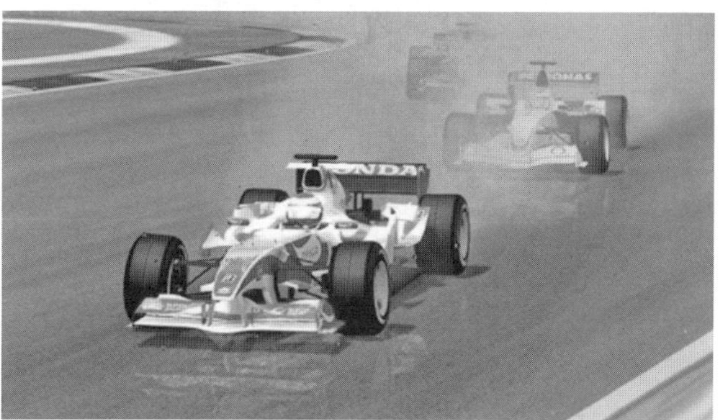

Fig. 31.2: Driving a race car is more visually demanding than everyday driving.

OCULOMOTOR SKILL

Saccades are more important than pursuits. Driver must be able to quickly and accurately locate landmarks, corner workers, pit crew and other disturbances that may arise. Pursuits are needed when the driver is watching his competition during practice from the sidelines, also while driving, to follow other driver's course line.

DEPTH PERCEPTION

Good depth perception for accurate steering judgement when approaching the apex of the corners is very important in car racing **(Fig. 31.3)**. Poor depth perception may lead to late braking, missing a wet patch on the track and missing braking points. Depth perception is also important considerations to integrate the information from peripheral awareness while overtaking other drivers.

BINOCULAR VISION

Binocular vision is very critical in car racing as it facilitates peripheral awareness and provides good depth perception. Good binocular vision becomes more demanding during the last few laps of the race when most attempts are made at passing and visual, mental and physical fatigue start affecting reaction time.

CENTRAL-PERIPHERAL AWARENESS

Central vision is needed to maintain a line or aiming. More than the central vision, peripheral vision is important for the drivers to be able to see other cars alongside of his own, and to be aware of the edges of the pavements.

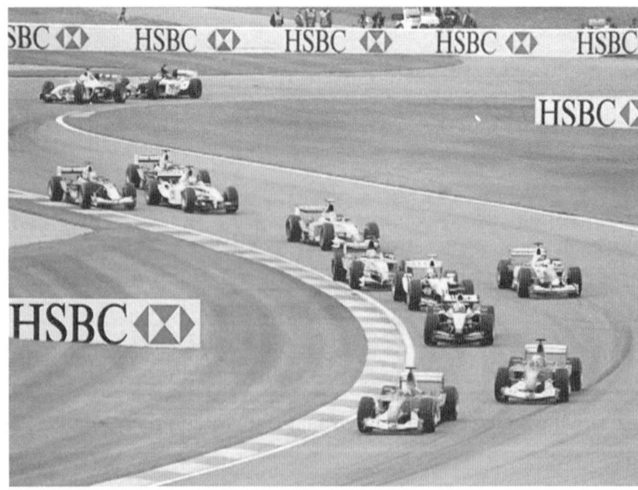

Fig. 31.3: Judgement of apex of the corners and relative distance of the other contestants needs good depth perception ability.

■ EYE-HAND-FOOT COORDINATION

Driver's ability to interpret visual input, and then successfully coordinate his hands and feet movement, is a key element in car racing. The driver must be able to make hand and foot movement for shifting and braking, after properly interpreting the visual stimulus. Although not purely visual, this could be the most important skill for a successful car driver. Faster reaction from the visual stimulus is very critical to prevent serious incidents.

■ GLARE RECOVERY

Glare recovery speed is not a very critical factor in car racing.

Driving is a visually sensitive sport. The eyes and vision are particularly susceptible to many external and internal factors. Externally carbon particles may cause watering and discomfort which lead to degraded vision, reduced concentration and mental fatigue. Internally the air in the cockpit is of particular concern as vision is more sensitive to air pollution. These factors will directly affect lap time and at worst they could lead to fatality. Visual performance in race drivers can be maximized by attention to:

- Peripheral awareness.
- Excessive head movement.
- Cockpit ventilation.
- Driver hydration/nutrition.
- Sudden auditory interruption.

Visual Demands in Downhill Skiing

32 CHAPTER

Downhill skiing is a recreational activity as well as a competitive sport. The sport involves sliding down snow covered hills with long, thin skis attached to each foot. The sport is popular wherever the combination of snow, mountain slopes, and a tourist infrastructure is available, including much of Europe, North America, and Japan. The sport is very fast and requires entire body balancing. The upper body remains more vertical than the lower body throughout the race and the hands are in front of the body to aid the balance. The secret of success lies simply into the ability of the skier to control the direction and speed of their descent. Typically, novice skiers use a technique called the "snow plough" to turn and stop by pointing one or both skis inward, but more advanced skiers use more difficult but more elegant and speedier method. As the skiers gain confidence, they tackle steeper, longer and more uneven slopes at higher speed. The speed, endurance and strength needed for the sport suggest it to be a dynamic event where good amount of physical control and balance are needed.

Atmospheric condition and the great speed involved in the sport make it a highly visually demanding sport. Both aiming and anticipation by depth perception are critical in downhill skiing. The skier's entire body weight should be predominantly on the downhill skiing while negotiating a turn, shoulder should remain horizontal, hands in front, poles aiming rearward and down, knees must be bent, the hip should be oriented uphill, while the shoulder and forearm are directed downhill and the eyes downhill steadily without any distraction, looking in the intended direction of travel **(Fig. 32.1)**. The entire body is controlled with respect to skis and the two poles which serve the purpose of alignment cues for aiming and is achieved with the help of peripheral awareness. Anticipation is needed for accurate turn. Poor anticipation may lead to either turning too quickly, causing overturning, or turn too slow, causing under turning. Anticipation is also needed to assess the relative distance and speed of the other contestants.

The importance of various elements of visual system in Downhill Skiing can be understood by following description:

VISUAL ACUITY

The visual acuity in downhill skiing is very much influenced by environmental hazards and is therefore, very critical. The skier must be able to see small objects in the terrain that might present a hazard such as rocks, tree branches, stumps and bare spots. The ability to read signs of marked trails, snow

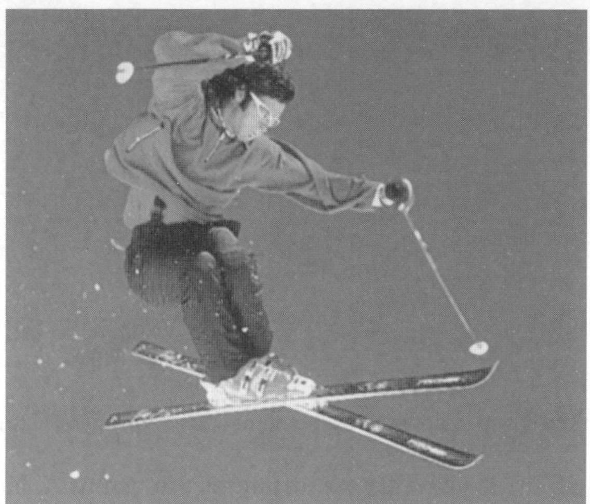

Fig. 32.1: Adventurous downhill skiing.

conditions, changing weather pattern are important ability in skiing safely and preventing a health hazard. These may be common to an experienced skier or may seem like common sense, but many new comers to skiing sport get lost on a mountain or suffer from hypothermia for failing to respond to posted changing conditions. Nature is dynamic, and skiing requires visual information for good judgement. Objects—especially other skiers, appear smaller, as they are farther away as you stand at the top of a ski trail. Discerning between people in front of you and those in between the path is necessary for safe and under-control skiing. All these are important elements while the skier is in motion, hence dynamic visual acuity is more important than static visual acuity and as the speed increases, the demand for this skill increases **(Fig. 32.2)**. Visual acuity is the function of contrast sensitivity. Poor contrast may affect visual acuity. Without good contrast sensitivity, you are at the mercy of the hill when the light goes flat and you cannot spot treacherous terrain before it swallows you up. Research shows wearing the right correction in a suitable filter can enhance the ability to see and distinguish the details especially in flat lighting conditions. Although color perception is not a major factor in skiing, distinguishing between certain colors may become difficult in a particular lighting condition. Caution should be taken while selecting the sunglasses that they do not distort color perception.

ACCOMMODATION–VERGENCE FUNCTION

Fast sports require fast eyes. Shifting of focus from far to near, from optical infinity to ten feet, must be efficient. Static focusing does not allow efficient or pretty skiing. As the skier becomes aware of the terrain in front and at the gates, other skiers and trees, slow shifting of focus delays processing for quick decision making. The demand for accommodation and vergence increases with higher speed and more difficult terrain. Together with speed of focusing,

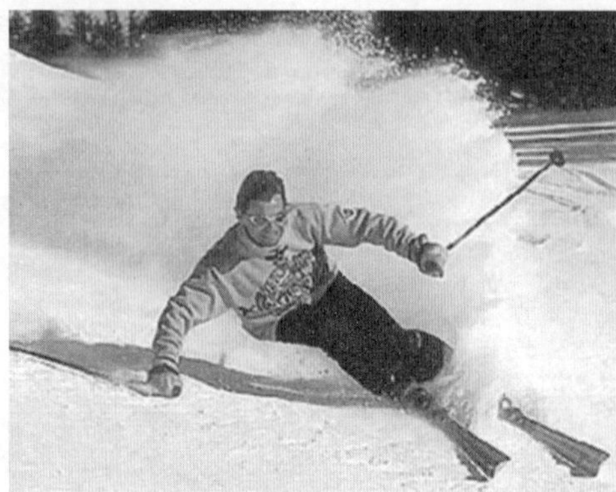

Fig. 32.2: The speed in downhill skiing demands good dynamic visual acuity.

fast fusional ability is also very important as the two work hand in hand, affecting the skier's overall performance.

OCULOMOTOR SKILL

Saccadic fixation is critical during the downhill skiing, skiing through trees, and around gates. Pursuits are used in following the other skiers down the mountain. Fixation is needed to maintain direction through the terrain.

DEPTH PERCEPTION

Depth perception ability is important to anticipate the distance between objects and the relative distance and speed of the other competitors. It is also critical while making turn. Poor depth perception may lead to either turning too quickly, causing overturning, or turn too slow. Although monocular depth cues are available, stereopsis aids the skiers in processing visual information about depth when monocular cues are sometimes absent.

BINOCULAR VISION

Every visual skill including binocular vision is very essential in skiing to maintain attention and concentration because of the high probability health hazards including the risk of death. Binocular vision improves visual acuity, provides depth perception ability, widens peripheral vision and facilitates contrast sensitivity—all of which are very important in skiing. Binocular vision also stops the muscles around the eyes from getting tired which may affect the performance during the last stages of the competition.

CENTRAL-PERIPHERAL AWARENESS

The high visual acuity demand makes central vision very important skill to look where the skier is going in front and to maintain the correct direction.

Good peripheral awareness is critical in keeping the skier safe from the whole field and to maintain body balance and seeing others in your field of vision. Central-peripheral awareness in skiing is one of the most important element of visual needs as it affects both aiming and anticipation during the event **(Fig. 32.3)**.

EYE-HAND-BODY COORDINATION

Serious athletes know how important their eyesight is. They know that they must work to enhance their eye-hand-body coordination **(Fig. 32.4)**. Good coordination starts with good vision. Eye-hand-body coordination is the way your hands, feet, body and muscles react to the information gathered by the eyes. The eyes determine speed, timing and mind-body control. When split seconds can make all the difference in performance and safety, speed of reaction is crucial. In skiing speed of reaction skill is used to make decisions about terrain hazards in an effort to avoid them and permits the redirection of body and skis almost simultaneously.

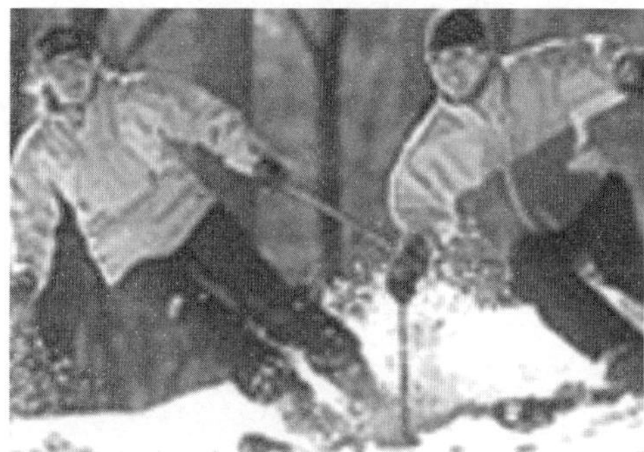

Fig. 32.3: Critical peripheral awareness for safe navigation in skiing

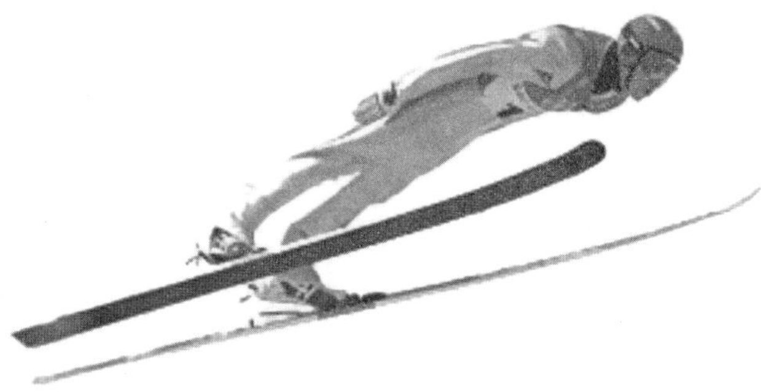

Fig. 32.4: Imagine the demand for excellent eye-hand-body coordination in skiing.

GLARE RECOVERY

Bright sunlight and glare from the snow are particularly demanding and takes its toll on skiers mentally and physically. In addition to the decreased visual performance, prolonged exposure to bright sunlight and ultraviolet rays can precipitate the formation of cataract. However, during the explosive moment of speed and turn, the glare may stun the skier and may cause accidents. Therefore, fast glare recovery is very important in skiing.

Visual efficiency is very important in downhill skiing as it will directly affect reaction time, balance, eye-hand-body coordination, which can make a difference between a good and a great run. Visualization is also plays an important part in the ability of a skier. Unable to visualize at the high altitude may often lead to panic attack.

Ocular Injuries in Sports

33 CHAPTER

According to American Academy of Ophthalmology, more than 40,000 eye injuries are caused by sports and recreational activities **(Fig. 33.1)**. The number only reflects those that were reported, but the actual estimates may be to the tune of 1,00,000. Most of these eye injuries are preventable. Studies show that 90% of sports related eye injuries are preventable. The sad part about eye injuries is that they often result in permanent damage. Many athletes have lost their careers due to an eye injury. The eyes are probably the most important part of the body needed to compete effectively in sports. However, most people do not take any measure to protect them. They protect their heads with helmets and their body with pads, but few eyewear to protect their eyes.

There are many factors that increase the risk of injury. Those with low skill levels, often found in the younger athletes, are at greater risk. Therefore, the young children should be protected, as any eye injury could permanently end their future in sport. Also those with pre-existing weak eye condition are at a bigger risk. For instance, if an athlete is playing with low vision in one eye and good vision in another, precaution should be taken to protect the good eye, as any injury to good eye could result in vision loss, reducing overall vision of the athlete. Also, those with high prescription may be at a bigger risk for permanent damage due to the inherent weakness pre-existing in their eyes

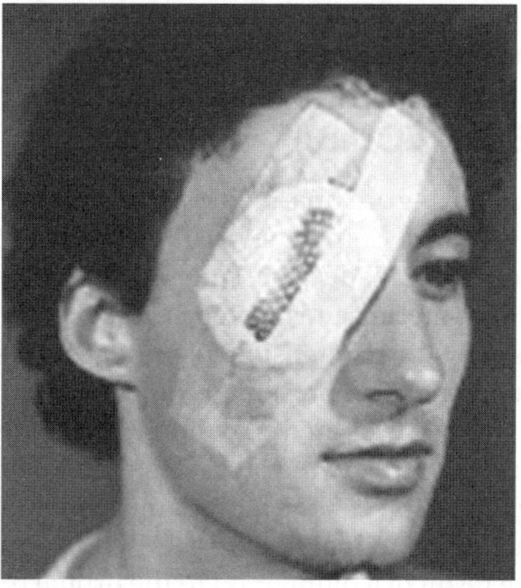

Fig. 33.1: Ocular injury in sports.

and those who had eye surgery may also be at a greater risk, since surgery may have weakened the natural state of the eye. Another factor that increases the risk of eye injury is the type of sport. Athletes participating in fast dynamic sports are more prone to ocular injuries than the athletes participating in non-dynamic slow sports.

EYE INJURIES IN RACQUET SPORTS

Tennis, squash, badminton are common racquet sports and all of them have very high velocity projectile, squash ball being the fastest moving sport. Shuttlecock in badminton can also attain a velocity of 135 mph. Both racquet and ball can cause injury. Possibility of injury increases in doubles as the two players occupy the place in the same court. Approximately one-half of the eye injuries from racquet sports are inflicted by the racquet itself. This type of blunt injury frequently results in ocular contusion at the site of impact. In most patients, the impact is on the cornea or the limbus, causing damage to the underlying vascular tissues. This can lead to bleeding into the anterior chamber of the eye and is called a hyphema. After the initial pain associated with the impact, a dull ache continues for several hours. Vision may be markedly reduced, but will improve as the hyphema (blood clot) settles. Occasionally, there may be some bleeding of the white of the eye. This looks quite alarming, but represents exterior bleeding which is not nearly as consequential as interior bleeding. Shuttlecock and the squash ball can penetrate the orbital cavity, causing serious eye trauma. In a survey of eye injury in sports, squash was considered to be the most dangerous in terms of risk of eye injury. Most of the eye injuries are caused by the ball. The classical risk situation is a player caught at the front of the court, turning to watch the progress of his shot, being hit by opponent's next stroke. Injuries in racquet sports can easily be prevented through the use of sport goggles. These goggles not only provide protection from injury, but can also be fitted with your prescription in them. Even if you need a slight vision correction, it will help you see the ball one second sooner, or help your aim by a fraction of an inch.

EYE INJURIES IN COMBAT SPORTS

Wrestling, judo, and boxing are unarmed combat sports that aim to simulate or cause injury **(Fig. 33.2)**. Combat sports frequently experience scratched and abraded corneas from inadvertent finger pokes. These are very painful, irritating and result in watering and blurred vision. Boxing among the combat sports is clearly played with an intension to injure, with loss of consciousness of the opponent being the most prestigious objective. Although protected by very hard bone on the side eyes are very vulnerable to direct hits from below. Damage to the eyes in boxing can result from direct contact or from shock waves. Depending on the force of the blow damage may result in injury to the retina, retinal detachment, retinal hemorrhage, etc. Contusion of the eyelids which is usually the result of a blunt or hit to the orbital margin or eyelids are

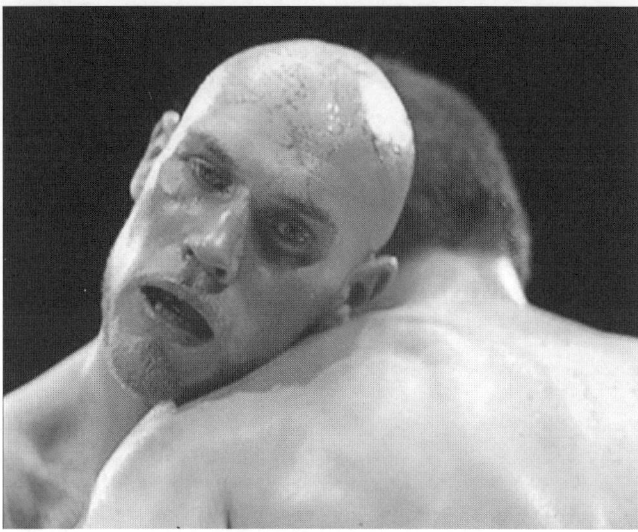

Fig. 33.2: Ocular injury in boxing.

quite common in boxing. The armed combat sports require body protection. At times failure to either the weapon or the protection may occur. In 1982, orbital penetration was reported due to broken fencing blade passed through the facemask of an international fencer.

EYE INJURIES IN BAT AND STICK SPORTS

Cricket, hockey, baseball, golf are some of the popular different bat and ball sports **(Fig. 33.3)**, but they share certain common characteristics. The projectile is small, hard and travels at a high velocity when struck by either a bat or a club. The ball is struck when it is in motion except golf in which the ball is struck by the club when it is static. Study shows that in hockey most of the injuries are caused by hockey stick. Hyphema, and orbital fracture are most commonly reported ocular injuries which can be produced by opponent's stick. Cricket batsman are more at risk than the bowlers. Ruptured globe, retinal detachment, hyphemas and lid laceration are common ocular injuries. However, many cricket batsmen now wear protective head helmets through which the ball cannot get onto the eye. Although golf injuries are rare, golf balls can produce very serious injuries. Golf ball and club both can fit within the bony orbit and result in globe trauma followed by enucleation and globe ruptured. Due to severity of golf related ocular injury, eye protection should always be considered and emphasized by the practitioners.

EYE INJURIES IN LARGE BALL SPORTS

Large ball sports are usually fast moving sports and involve handling of ball. Football, basketball, volleyball, rugby **(Fig. 33.4)**, handball are most popular

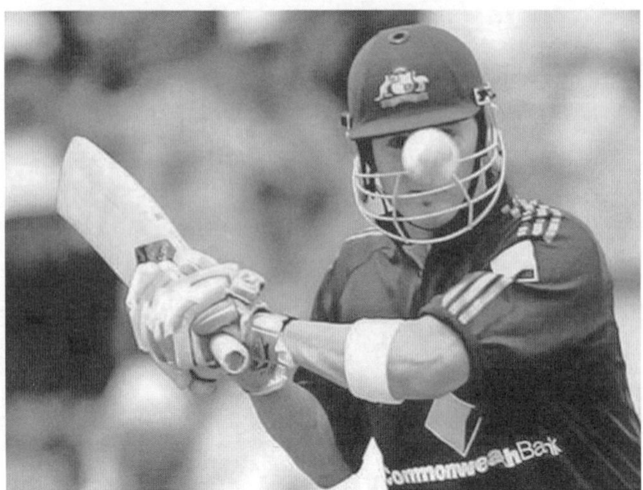

Fig. 33.3: Possibility of eye injury in cricket.

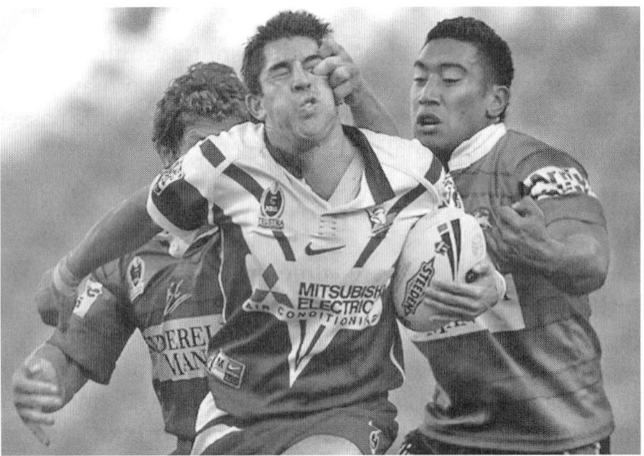

Fig. 33.4: Eye gouge in rugby.

among them. Although the ball is always in motion, it is not the major cause of ocular injuries. The hard shot striking the head may have partial penetration into the orbit, but such injuries are rare. Physical clashes with opponent's hands , elbows, feet or sometimes fists can hit eyes accidentally and can cause injury to the eyes. Such injuries are typically seen in basketball, and rugby. Deliberate hit with hands are quite common in rugby. That is why widespread use of helmets are quite common in rugby.

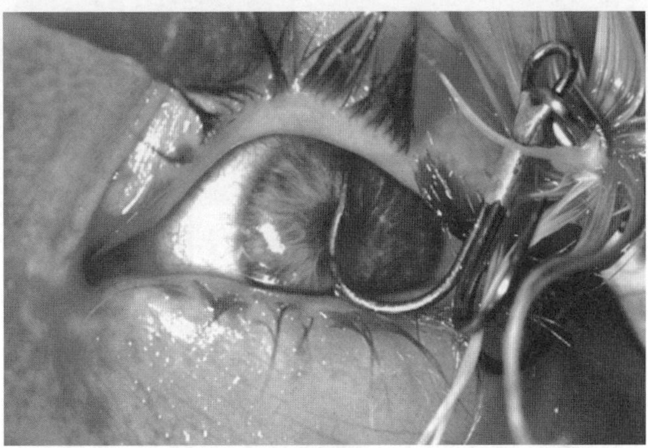

Fig. 33.5: Fishing hook in the left eye.

EYE INJURIES IN WATER SPORTS

Swimming, yachting, fishing and scuba diving are most popular among the water sports. Prolonged exposure to chlorine in pools can start to eat away the corneal surface of the eye. Ill-fitted or badly handled swimming goggle may cause injuries to the eyes. Over-tightening of goggles may cause swollen eyelids. Vision loss has been reported after elasticized goggle were pulled away from the face, slipped from the hand and recoiled with the great force into the face. Fishing injuries, particularly from hooks **(Fig. 33.5)** are serious and can result in enucleation. During scuba diving , the relative changes of the environmental pressure are transmitted to the eyes and the periocular tissue-barotraumas occurs when there is a loss of pressure equilibrium. Diving may be hazardous for the patients who have undergone ocular surgery. There is a theoretical possibility of corneal rupture in divers following refractive surgery.

EYE INJURIES IN SNOW SPORTS

Snow sports are fast and dynamic sports. Skiing and ice-hockey are most popular. High altitude exposure can cause hypoxia which can lead to increased retinal blood flow, resulting into the predisposition to intraretinal hemorrhage. The loss of an eye has been reported because of stick coming in between face and face protector in ice-hockey. Puck may also cause ocular injury **(Fig. 33.6)**.

SUMMARY

Studies shows that ocular injuries resulting from modern sports are often severe. Many athletes argue that they have never suffered any eye injury, and neither have any close acquaintances. That is why they do not need any eye protection. The authors would like to point out that accidents do not happen regularly and when they happen, they do not give alert signals. At times, it

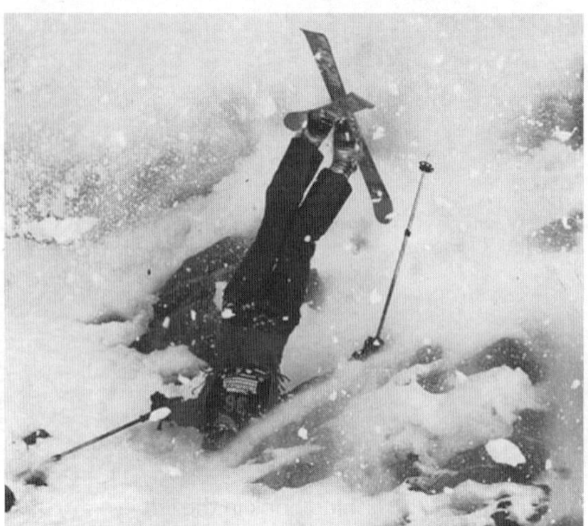

Fig. 33.6: Possible injury in skiing.

may not be because of any mistake on the part of the athlete, nor because of opponent. It is a matter of appreciating the probability of risks and making sensible judgments to enhance the sporting life of an athlete. However, considering the severity of ocular injury sustained during the sport it has been argued that adequate instruction of the participants in the game, proper use of eye protectors, and a complete ophthalmological examination after an eye trauma should be mandatory.

Setting up the Sport Vision Practice

34 CHAPTER

Sport vision optometry represents a specialized branch within the field of optometry, aimed at enhancing athletic performance through vision optimization. Despite its potential, the field faces challenges in gaining widespread acceptance.

FACTORS HINDERING ACCEPTANCE

Several factors contribute to this, including limited awareness, research, and professional resources.

Limited Awareness

Many athletes, coaches, clubs and institutes are not aware of the benefits of sports vision training and its potential impact on athletic performance. The lack of awareness hinders the adoption of sports vision optometry. Greater education and outreach efforts are needed to highlight the advantages of sport vision services.

Limited Research

The scientific understanding of sports vision and its impact on performance is still developing. Increased research funding and collaboration can further elucidate the role of vision in athletics.

Lack of Expert Professionals

There is a shortage of optometrists and vision therapists with specialized training in sportvision. One of the biggest differences between sport vision practice and general optometry practice is while the general optometry can be set up without a team of people other than clerical staffs, for sport vision practice there is a need of a team of specialized personnel who are trained in vision therapy and in one or more of vision enhancement activities especially for full grown practice.

Lack of Professional Referral System

A formalized referral system between optometrists, coaches, and sports teams is absent. Building networks and partnerships within the sporting community can facilitate referrals to sport vision practitioners.

Lack of Resource Materials

Comprehensive educational materials and guidelines for sportvision practice are limited. Developing standardized protocols and resources can support practitioners in delivering effective services.

Limited Educational Institutions

Few institutions offer specialized education and training in sportvision services. Expanding curriculum offerings and training opportunities can foster the development of skilled professionals.

Emphasis on Product Sales

Some sport vision practices prioritize selling aids over comprehensive assessments and follow-ups. Shifting focus towards holistic vision care and performance enhancement strategies is essential.

Absence of Recognized Certification

There is no universally recognized certification program for sportvision practitioners. Establishing accreditation standards can ensure competency and quality of care within the field.

Cost of Advanced Tools

Advanced diagnostic tools for sport vision assessment can be prohibitively expensive. Efforts to make equipment more affordable and accessible can lower barriers to entry for practitioners.

FEATURES OF A SPORT VISION PRACTICE

The primary distinction between sport vision practice and other forms of optometry lies in the nature of the relationship between the practitioner and the individual seeking care. In traditional optometry, the dynamic is characterized by a patient-practitioner relationship, whereas in sportvision practice, it centers around an athlete-practitioner relationship. In general optometry practice, patients typically seek assistance when encountering difficulties in seeing objects either at a distance, up close, or experiencing various visual symptoms. Optometrists conduct examinations using high-contrast Snellen's charts in an ideally lit room with static conditions and ample visual stimuli. Following assessment, optometrists prescribe corrective measures enabling patients to achieve clear vision, often targeting the 20/20 or 6/6 line on the chart. Alternatively, patients may undergo examinations using a slit lamp, where optometrists diagnose conditions, search for pertinent signs related to symptoms, and if necessary, refer them to ophthalmologists for specialized treatment. In this setting, patients generally play a passive role, receiving expert guidance and recommendations from optometrists who lead the consultation and carry out necessary procedures.

The practice of sport vision differs significantly from traditional optometry. In sport vision, athletes are not treated as patients since they typically possess healthier visual systems compared to the general population. Instead of diagnosing eye diseases or providing ocular treatments, sport vision practitioners focus on evaluating the athlete's visual function comprehensively. Unlike a standard eye examination, the sport vision examiner doesn't aim to diagnose or treat eye conditions. Rather, they meticulously assess the athlete's visual function, record the findings, and analyze the data. The goal is to identify any deficiencies that may impact the athlete's sporting performance. This analysis incorporates the practitioner's understanding of the specific demands of the athlete's sport. Following assessment, the sport vision practitioner collaborates with the athlete and their coach to develop an action plan aimed at enhancing sporting performance by addressing any identified visual deficiencies. This process is not typically completed in a single session, as ongoing evaluation and intervention are often necessary. Critical to the success of sportvision services is the active engagement of the athlete. Their input, along with that of their coach, is integral to tailoring interventions and ensuring their effectiveness within the context of the athlete's training regimen. Thus, sportvision examination serves as the starting point for a continuous process aimed at optimizing the athlete's visual performance and overall athletic abilities.

Some of the distinctive characteristics of sportvision practice can be studied as under:

Practice Objective

The primary objective of a sport vision clinic is to enhance sporting performance by optimizing the visual capabilities of athletes. This involves providing personalized interventions following preliminary consultations, fostering collaboration with coaches and trainers, ensuring continuity of care, and conducting periodic assessments to track progress. By prioritizing these objectives, a sport vision clinic aims to help athletes reach their full potential and excel in their respective sports.

Specialized Team

In sport vision practice, there is a need for a specialized team comprising individuals trained in vision therapy and various enhancement techniques tailored for athletes. Unlike a general optometry setting, a sportvision practice requires a dedicated team consisting of professionals such as optometrists specializing in sports vision, vision therapists, and technicians proficient in operating advanced equipment.

Collaborative Approach

A sport vision practice frequently collaborates with coaches, trainers, and sports medicine experts to enhance athlete performance. This collaborative approach ensures a comprehensive strategy for addressing visual factors affecting athletic success. With a focus on athlete-centered care, interventions are customized to meet each individual's unique visual demands. This may include personalized training plans, specialized eyewear recommendations, or tailored vision therapy programs.

Comprehensive Services

A comprehensive sportvision practice should provide a variety of services, encompassing screening, in-clinic assessments, and post-assessment therapies. Furthermore, the practice should be equipped with facilities for dispensing specialized sports eyewear, including spectacles and contact lenses tailored to enhance athletic performance.

SETTING UP THE SPORT VISION PRACTICE

Starting a sport vision practice can range from basic considerations such as eye dominance and color preference to a comprehensive practice offering screening, in-clinic assessments, and post-assessment therapies, including dispensing spectacles and contact lenses. Screening programs may be conducted in-clinic or on-site to identify visual deficiencies and factors limiting athletic performance.

A full grown sport vision practice should have all the tests needed to conduct an effective screening program not only at clinic but also at the site. The following set of equipment needed to organize an effective sports vision screening program:

- High and low LogMAR charts
- Brock string
- Dynamic fixation
- Howell Phoria test
- TNO stereopsis
- Retinoscope
- Color preference test
- Ocular dominance
- Stop watch
- Lux meter
- Measuring tap
- Station posters
- Clipboard

In addition, Basin Anticipation Timer may be added to the above list.

After the screening process, a detailed report containing statistical analysis including mean, standard deviation, and individual vision profiles should be submitted to the club's authority. Athletes identified with visual deficiencies should be referred to a sports vision clinic for a comprehensive examination. A fully equipped sports vision clinic should also possess the following additional equipment:

- ❖ Mallet unit for distance
- ❖ Mallet unit for near
- ❖ Duochrome test
- ❖ Trial Lens set
- ❖ Ishihara color vision test
- ❖ Fanchart
- ❖ High contrast Snellen's chart
- ❖ Basin Anticipation timer
- ❖ Dynamic Vision rotator
- ❖ Contrast Sensitivity Tester CVS 1000
- ❖ Wayne Saccadic Fixator
- ❖ Acuvision 1000
- ❖ Peripheral awareness test

Having these additional tools ensures a comprehensive evaluation and treatment approach for athletes with visual deficiencies, allowing for tailored interventions to optimize their performance.

SETTING UP THE FEES STRUCTURE

Sports vision practice is a specialized field within optometry that requires careful consideration of revenue models from the outset. Various practice models exist, each requiring a tailored fee structure. For instance, in an independent clinic setup, professional fees can be based on hours of engagement per visit, with initial consultations charged slightly higher than follow-up appointments. Office-based sports vision therapy may be charged at standard rates, either daily or as part of a program, with additional charges for appliances like contact lenses or protective goggles invoiced separately.

Retainer fees can vary based on the practitioner's credentials and level of involvement, though this model may require availability at short notice. Screening programs necessitate a separate financial strategy, which could involve funding through the clinic's marketing budget or sponsorship. If a sports club expresses interest in vision training for their athletes, negotiations can be initiated based on the practitioner's expertise and credentials. Overall, establishing a robust revenue model ensures sustainability and viability for the sports vision practice.

The Future of Sports Vision

35 CHAPTER

Sports have served as a crucial avenue for individuals to hone their skills and navigate societal changes. Throughout history, sports have reflected shifts in social dynamics and human endeavors. From rural games transitioning to urban centers during the industrial revolution to the globalization of sports rules and professionalism, the evolution of sports mirrors broader societal transformations.

In the contemporary landscape, sports participation is widely regarded as a means to enhance physical fitness and overall well-being. The sports industry has burgeoned into one of the largest worldwide, with millions of individuals engaging in sports and leisure activities. Athletes at the elite level command star status, attracting significant investments in advertising, sponsorship, and professional fees.

Looking ahead, the future of sports vision promises significant changes driven by advancements in media, technology, and athlete analysis. The proliferation of media channels and internet platforms, coupled with sophisticated technology, will revolutionize how athletes' abilities are assessed and optimized.

Governing bodies and forward-thinking practitioners will seize the opportunity to embrace these changes, while others risk obsolescence. The future of sports vision will prioritize every aspect contributing to an athlete's performance, including visual skills.

Athletes are increasingly cognizant of the intense competition in sports and the critical role of physical fitness in their careers. They recognize the importance of optimal eye protection and high-level visual skills for peak performance.

Sports vision specialists, adept at prescribing and dispensing eyewear tailored to specific sports, will play a pivotal role in enhancing athletes' visual acuity and overall performance. These specialists will collaborate with athletes to optimize their visual capabilities, providing essential services for achieving success in sports.

The historical progression of vision correction underscores the significance of vision care in enhancing athletic performance. From early spectacles to modern contact lenses and laser surgery, advancements in vision correction have been integral to improving visual acuity.

The establishment of sports vision as a distinct discipline within optometry reflects the growing recognition of its importance in sports performance. Research conducted by organizations like Sportvision Ltd, underscores the urgent need for optometric services to support athletes in achieving Olympic success.

Despite the exponential growth of sports participation, the development of sports vision practice has not fully mirrored this trend. Many eye care professionals remain unaware of the sports vision needs of their patients and the potential for practice growth in this area.

In countries like UK and USA, efforts to understand the role of vision in sports performance have led to the establishment of sports vision associations and specialized training programs. However, in countries like India, where significant investments are made in sports, there remains untapped potential for leveraging vision training to enhance athlete performance.

The future of sports vision holds promise for interdisciplinary collaboration between eyecare professionals, sports authorities, and manufacturers. Individual and team sports may appoint dedicated sports vision consultants, akin to trainers and coaches, to optimize visual performance.

By embracing the evolving landscape of sports vision, practitioners can gain a competitive edge and contribute to the holistic development of athletes. Proactive engagement with new developments in sports vision will pave the way for innovation and advancement in the field, ultimately benefiting athletes and sports enthusiasts worldwide.

Multiple Choice Questions

1. **What is expected of vision assessment as far as sports vision practice is concerned?**
   a. The athlete needs to understand that visual assessment will never make things worse, but potential for improvement is enormous.
   b. The athlete needs to understand that visual assessment will provide them an extra edge over others that most athletes are looking for today at the elite level.
   c. The athlete needs to understand that sports vision optometry is based on the concept that eyes are also the part of same physiological system as other bodily functions. If one of the bodily functions does not work properly, it will have effect on other bodily functions too.
   d. All of the above.

2. **Why are visual clues important in sports?**
   a. Early pick up of visual clues helps precise anticipation and thereby provides extra time to respond.
   b. Visual clues helps maintain alignment and direction in accordance with the need of the sporting event.
   c. Both of the above.
   d. None of the above.

3. **Which of the following statements is correct with respect to visual clues in sports?**
   a. Pattern of wind on water provides clues to the direction and intensity of air and thus helps in yachting to make tactical decision.
   b. Speed and direction of racket helps the opponent in table tennis to anticipate shot type.
   c. Both of the above.
   d. Only (b) is correct.

4. **Which of the following is most appropriate about vision as far as sports vision optometry is concerned?**
   a. Vision implies seeing last line clearly in the test chart.
   b. Vision implies taking the information and initiating the appropriate response.
   c. Vision implies that the athletes should be able to aim at the target accurately.
   d. All of the above.

5. **Which one of the following is the symptom of visual stress?**
   a. Discomfort while reading
   b. Continually losing the place on the page or skipping lines
   c. Sensations of text moving on the page or screen
   d. All of the above
6. **Which of the following factors influence the overall visual demand in a given sport?**
   a. Target size and distance
   b. Speed of the target and speed of athletes
   c. Ambient light levels and position of luminaries
   d. All of the above
7. **Which of the following visual skill is critical in sailing?**
   a. Eye movement
   b. Peripheral awareness
   c. Glare recovery
   d. All of the above
8. **Which of the following is more relevant statement with respect to cricket?**
   a. Anticipation is more important in batting and aiming is dominating element in bowling.
   b. Eye movement is important in batting and peripheral awareness is important in fielding.
   c. Fast eyes are associated with cricket.
   d. None of the above.
9. **Which of the following is the important precursor to fixation?**
   a. Good foveal function and the object must have attention value.
   b. Move and get in the right position to fixate
   c. Precise stereoscopic vision.
   d. None of the above.
10. **Which of the following sport is predominantly aiming sports?**
   a. Rifle shooting
   b. Tennis
   c. Golf
   d. Cricket
11. **If an athlete cannot maintain steady fixation what could be the possible reason?**
   a. Fatigue
   b. Drug effects
   c. Congenital nystagmus
   d. All of the above

12. The ability to anticipate is the function of:

a. Depth perception
b. Contrast sensitivity
c. Accommodation
d. Eye movement

13. Quick and accurate anticipation relies heavily on

a. How quickly and accurately the athlete picks up the visual clues.
b. Good Visual Acuity
c. Fast Eye Movement
d. None of the above

14. Which of the following sports is predominantly anticipatory?

a. Rifle Shooting
b. Cricket
c. Tennis
d. Golf

15. Which of the following sports combine both aiming and anticipation?

a. Golf
b. Cricket
c. Tennis
d. Rifle Shooting

16. Which of the following is the primary visual skill in sports?

a. Aiming
b. Visual Acuity
c. Fixation Disparity
d. Color Preference

17. What is the likely proportion of the primary visual skills—aiming and anticipation in snooker?

a. 20:80
b. 50:50
c. 60:40
d. 80:20

18. The ability to judge the distance and speed of approach of a moving object requires:

a. Active accommodation and good vergence facility
b. Visual acuity and binocular coordination
c. Good contrast
d. All of the above

19. In table tennis a good anticipation includes:

a. Anticipating the ball trajectory
b. Direction of opponent's stroke

c. Temporal judgment of environment and opponent's pattern of play
d. All of the above

20. Which of the following is true regarding aiming in sports?

a. While aiming generally there is an alignment
b. Dominant eye facilitates aiming
c. Central-peripheral awareness is very critical for aiming
d. All of the above

21. Which sport shows a good balance between aiming and anticipation?

a. Snooker
b. Tennis
c. Archery
d. Football

22. Which is the most important visual skill for reading?

a. Aiming
b. Anticipation
c. Depth perception
d. Accommodation

23. What is visual acuity?

a. Visual acuity is the time dependent measurement of retinal health, specified by the date.
b. Vision with spectacle
c. Vision with contact lenses
d. All of the above

24. The visual acuity is not dependent upon:

a. Pupil size
b. Spherical aberration
c. Chromatic aberration
d. Corneal refractive index

25. What is the normal viewing distance for measuring visual acuity on Snellen's test chart?

a. 1 m
b. 2 m
c. 4 m
d. 6 m

26. Which of the following is more relevant in sport as far as visual acuity is concerned?

a. Visual acuity affects the ability to pick up on visual clues.
b. The derivation is if you can see the target clearly, you can fixate at the same.

   c. Good visual acuity implies good foveal vision which is extremely important for aiming in sports.
   d. All of the above.

27. Which of the following is more relevant of measuring vernier acuity in sports vision practice?
   a. Vernier acuity also known as hyper acuity, measures the accuracy with which the subject can judge whether targets are aligned or not.
   b. Though vernier acuity is not a diagnostic measure of visual performance, it opens up the scope for discussion when the athlete finds that his Vernier acuity is significantly reduced.
   c. It corresponds to recognition of relative position.
   d. None of the above.

28. Which of the following is correct for dynamic visual acuity?
   a. Dynamic visual acuity worsens rapidly with age
   b. Females have slightly higher dynamic visual acuity than males.
   c. Dynamic visual acuity and static visual acuity are same in most subjects.
   d. All of the above.

29. Which of the following clinical situations will not reduce contrast sensitivity while visual acuity may remain same?
   a. Capsular opacification of lenses
   b. Corneal edema
   c. Oxidative changes due to heavy smoking
   d. None of the above.

30. A steady dominant eye is important:
   a. To hold the visual system steady at the fixating target.
   b. To enable the athlete to see the target more clearly.
   c. To prevent the eyes from fatigue.
   d. None of the above.

31. What happens when natural ocular dominance is disturbed?
   a. It may lead to attention jump while reading.
   b. Binocular instability may occur.
   c. The athlete may not be able to hold the fixation at the target for long.
   d. All of the above.

32. Which of the following is *not* true regarding dominant eye?
   a. Dominant eye is the fixating eye in the binocular vision.
   b. Dominant eye aims at the object.
   c. Dominant eye leads in receiving the visual inputs.
   d. Dominant eye is the eye with better visual acuity.

33. The ability to judge the distance and speed of approach of a moving object requires:

a. Active accommodation and good vergence facility.

b. Visual acuity and binocular coordination.

c. Good contrast.

d. All of the above.

34. Depth judgement affects

a. Making spatial judgment of the ball

b. Making judgment regarding the speed of approaching ball

c. Making judgment regarding direction of the arriving ball

d. All of the above

35. Poor depth judgement ability can be effectively treated with:

a. Refractive error correction

b. Vision therapy

c. Proper diet and nutrition

d. All of the above

36. Which of the following is the progenitor of depth judgment?

a. Fusion

b. Fixation

c. Suppression

d. Vergence

37. The slightly different images a person's two eyes send to the brain is known as:

a. Motion parallax

b. Retinal disparity

c. Relative size

d. Linear perspective

38. Monocular depth cues include all of the following, *except*:

a. Relative size

b. Convergence

c. Interposition

d. Linear perspective

39. Which of the following is *correct* regarding depth perception?

a. Correcting depth perception problems may be as simple as correcting a refractive error so that both eyes have the same visual acuity.

b. Vision therapy is one of the ways to treat depth perception issues.

c. Rolling the eyes, shifting eye gaze, resting the dominant eye may help improving the depth perception.

d. All of the above.

40. Which of the following is true about depth perception?

a. You need to have fusion first before you can have depth perception.

b. Depth perception also lets you determine how fast an object is coming towards you.

c. Depth perception relates to spatial judgement.

d. All of the above.

41. Which of the following sports is likely to have the greatest need for peripheral awareness?

a. Football

b. Snooker

c. Clay pigeon shooting

d. Table tennis

42. Which of the following is true about peripheral awareness?

a. Peripheral awareness is the ability to be aware of peripheral objects while maintaining central vision.

b. Peripheral awareness is not only necessary to prepare you to react in time for objects and people that are approaching you from sides but also for your own safety.

c. Deficits can cause athletes to miss objects on the sides or be distracted by movement and objects in the peripheral field of vision.

d. All of the above.

43. Which of the following statement is *true* regarding peripheral awareness?

a. Peripheral awareness is the ability to see action or objects that are not in the direct line of vision.

b. Any deficit in peripheral awareness may cause athletes to be destructed by the movement and objects in the peripheral field of vision.

c. Peripheral awareness prepares an athlete to react in time.

d. All of the above.

44. Peripheral vision is reduced because of:

a. Increase in the speed of running

b. Because of glaucoma, strokes or head injury

c. With the increase in the degree of stress

d. All of the above.

45. Which of the followings is *not* the advantage of good peripheral vision?

a. Minimizes the possibility of injury

b. Improves anticipation

c. Increases reaction speed in athletes

d. Improves focusing ability of the athletes

46. Which skill is not measured by dynamic fixation?

a. Eye speed
b. Predisposition to athletic event
c. Hand-eye coordination
d. Event preparation

47. Human eye movement of back and forth during reading process in inquiry is defined as:

a. Saccades
b. Fixations
c. Suppression
d. Regressions

48. Which of the following is *not* correct for extraocular muscles?

a. EOMs are among the fastest muscles in human body.
b. EOMs are fatigue resistant.
c. EOMs need and receive more oxygen.
d. EOMs are inadequately supplied with blood vessels.

49. Which of the following is not true about saccades?

a. Saccades are fast eye movement.
b. Saccades shift the fixation abruptly.
c. Saccades redirect the line of sight so that the point of interest stimulates the fovea.
d. Saccades allow us to follow the moving object.

50. Which measurement can the Howell phoria test not do?

a. Fixation disparity
b. Vertical phorias
c. Peripheral awareness
d. All of the above

51. Which of the following is *not* correct?

a. During accommodation anterior surface of the lens becomes more convex
b. Pupil constricts
c. Central part of the iris advances, while the peripheral part recedes slightly
d. None of the above

52. Convergence insufficiency may make:

a. Things appear further away than actually they are
b. May result in loss of depth perception
c. May cause late breaking
d. All of the above

53. Which of the following is associated with close viewing distance?

a. The cilliary muscles contracts and in effect, reduces the tension that zonule exerts on the lens

b. The lens becomes more spherical and has greater refractive power

c. Pupil constricts

d. All of the above

54. What effect does not happen with convergence insufficiency in a Formula One racing driver?

a. Everything seems bigger

b. Late breaking

c. Things seems further away

d. More accidents happen when fatigued

55. Which is *least* important in a presbyopic pistol shooter?

a. Clear near sight

b. Clear target

c. Near addition

d. Larger shooting lens than a rifle shooter

56. Which of the following is the symptom of light sensitivity?

a. Rapid blinking, poor concentration, lowering of chin to shield the eyes

b. Narrowing of the palpebral aperture

c. Dark adaptation

d. All of the above

57. Which of the following behavior traits could be directly attributed to light sensitivity?

a. Poor attention in brightly lit classroom reading from a white page

b. Difficulty with overhead projectors

c. Severe disadvantages in outdoor sports

d. All of the above

58. Which of the following is *not* true?

a. A strong preference for blue tint and dislike of yellow tint indicates clinically significant light sensitivity.

b. A preference for yellow indicates no light sensitivity.

c. If all colors are equally liked, then it indicates no preference and good tolerance to color distortion and all colors are rejected, then it indicates intolerance to color distortion.

d. None of the above.

59. What is the main objective of sports vision assessment?

a. To examine the eyes and give them the appropriate lens prescription.

b. To elicit the ocular disorders and suggest a treatment plan.

c. To assess the visual system comprehensively, link the elements of the visual system to visual performance in the given sport and demonstrate how visual performance is affecting his sporting performance.
d. To examine the eye using most modern gadgets.

60. Which of the following is correct about retinoscopy?
a. It gives the initial view of the inside of the eye.
b. It helps to know the refractive status of the eye.
c. It is not dependent upon subject's response.
d. All of the above.

61. Which of the following is true about fixation disparity?
a. Fixation disparity is measured separately for distance and near.
b. Fixation disparity reduces level of stereopsis.
c. Prism is needed to correct the fixation disparity.
d. All of the above.

62. If refractive error is not fully corrected, it may lead to:
a. Either under or over accommodation.
b. Unusual demand of either negative or positive fusional vergence.
c. Decreased fusional ability as a result of blurred retinal images.
d. All of the above.

63. Which of the following situation during Brock string test determine the accuracy of binocular vision?
a. The two strings making cross at bead, i.e., object of regard.
b. The two strings appear to meet before the bead, i.e., object of regard.
c. The two strings appear to meet beyond the bead, i.e., beyond object of regard.
d. All of the above.

64. The reason suggested to have one or more of analytical test in the battery of sportvision test:
a. To diagnose the deficiency of the sporting skill.
b. To diagnose and demonstrate the deficiency of visual system.
c. There has to be a test for specific visual skill that has some reference to the specific skill of the given sport in which the athlete is specialized into, that can be used to test or screen a group of athletes and a comparative analytical study of their performance may be done to find out who needs full eye examination.
d. None of the above.

65. How can the sportvision optometrist design the appropriate analytical test for a given sport?
a. By reading sport vision books and find from there.
b. To pick up a test from the different set of tests that are already there in the consulting room.

c. A number of tests are available in real world and the practitioner can select any one out of those.
d. Analytical tests are ideally derived from the discussion with coaches and players within the club or from your own knowledge of sport.

66. What is the suggested criterion for selecting an appropriate analytical test?
a. It must be easy to perform.
b. It must represent the core sporting skill of the athlete.
c. It must affect or affected by at least two or more elements of visual skills that are listed in diagnostic tests.
d. It is a random selection.

67. Bassin Anticipation Timer is used to check:
a. Anticipation and eye-hand coordination
b. Aiming and dominant eye
c. Binocular coordination and visual acuity
d. All of the above

68. Poor performance on stereoacuity test represent:
a. Poor timing in executing shot
b. Poor aiming
c. Poor eye-hand coordination
d. Poor peripheral awareness

69. 'Ball catching' could be a good analytical tests in which of the following sports?
a. Cricket
b. Golf
c. Football
d. Hockey

70. Which of the following does not seem to be *true*?
a. Analytical tests can be derived from the discussion with coaches and players
b. Analytical tests can be derived from your own knowledge of sport
c. Analytical tests can be derived from your clinical experience and expertise
d. Analytical tests should be simple, repeatable and measurable objectively

71. Which of the following is *not* correct statement regarding dynamic sports?
a. Dynamic sports are explosive events.
b. Dynamic sports require high speed and energy.
c. Dynamic sports do not require control at all.
d. In dynamic sports things happen very quickly.

72. Which of the following sports is *not* non-dynamic sport?

a. Archery

b. Shooting

c. Yachting

d. Snooker

73. In which of the following sports near visual acuity does not affect sporting performance so much?

a. Golf

b. Snooker

c. Tennis

d. Cricket

74. Air contains how much percentage of oxygen:

a. 20.93%

b. 79.04%

c. 50%

d. 31.09%

75. Which of the following statement is incorrect?

a. As the altitude increases, the density of air decreases.

b. As the altitude increases, the partial pressure of oxygen decreases.

c. As the altitude increases, the effect of UV radiation decreases.

d. As the altitude increases, the temperature decreases.

76. Which of the following statement is *not true* about underwater environment?

a. The eyes become effectively myopic.

b. There is a selective absorption of light.

c. Objects appear larger.

d. There is lot of light scattering.

77. Which the following is the immediate effect of alcohol intake?

a. Dehydration

b. Reaction time, balance and coordination

c. Endurance and speed

d. All of the above

78. In which type of sport spectacle frames incorporating joints at or below the datum line that enables the wearer to see through the top portion of the lens in a leaning down position is useful?

a. Billiards

b. Table tennis

c. Chess

d. Rafting

79. Which of the following statement is *true*?

a. Yellow light focuses on the retina
b. Blue light focuses before retina
c. Red light focuses behind retina
d. All of the above

80. Which of the following is *not* an advantage of contact lenses?

a. Peripheral awareness
b. Normalized image size
c. Protection from trauma
d. Eliminates differential prisms

81. Which is the lens material of choice in sports lenses?

a. Quartz
b. CR 39
c. Polycarbonate
d. Toughened lenses

82. Which of the following is *not* associated with high base curve lenses?

a. Increase peripheral awareness
b. Increase dihedral angle
c. Small size lens
d. Recalculated lens power

83. Which of the following is *not* relevant to the sports frames?

a. Sports frames are flat across the front.
b. They have larger “A” measurement than “B” measurement.
c. They fit closer to the eyes compare to dress wear frames.
d. They are to be fitted with high curvature lenses.

ANSWERS

1. d	2. c	3. c	4. b	5. d	6. d	7. d	8. a	9. a	10. a
11. d	12. a	13. a	14. c	15. a	16. a	17. b	18. b	19. d	20. d
21. a	22. a	23. a	24. d	25. d	26. d	27. b	28. a	29. d	30. a
31. d	32. d	33. d	34. d	35. d	36. a	37. b	38. b	39. d	40. d
41. a	42. d	43. d	44. d	45. d	46. c	47. d	48. d	49. d	50. b
51. d	52. d	53. d	54. a	55. b	56. d	57. d	58. d	59. c	60. d
61. d	62. d	63. a	64. c	65. d	66. c	67. a	68. a	69. b	70. c
71. c	72. c	73. a	74. a	75. c	76. a	77. d	78. a	79. d	80. c
81. c	82. c	83. a							

79. Which of the following statement is true?
   a. Yellow light focuses on the retina
   b. Blue light focuses before retina
   c. Red light focuses behind retina
   d. All of the above
80. Which of the following is not an advantage of contact lenses?
   a. Peripheral awareness
   b. Normalized image size
   c. Protection from trauma
   d. Eliminates differential prisms
81. Which is the lens material of choice in sports lenses?
   a. Quartz
   b. Glass
   c. Polycarbonate
   d. [illegible]

[illegible]

Bibliography

1. Bob Decot. Old Pistol Shooters Don't Give Up, They Just Lose Their Sights.
2. Gerald E Lowther. Contact Lenses: Procedures and Techniques.
3. Geraint Griffiths. Eye Speed, Motility and Athletic Potential.
4. Ozzie Jacobs. What is the Meaning of Lifestyle?
5. Vince Lombardi. 5 Areas: Sleep has the Greatest Impact on Athletic Performance.
6. Brooke De Lench. Physical Abuse in Youth Sports Can Leave Emotional Scars.
7. Carla Hannaford. The Dominance Factor.
8. Geraint Griffiths. Eye Dominance in Sports: A Comparative Study.
9. Jonathan S Pointer. Sighting versus Sensory Ocular Dominance.
10. Siofra Harrington. A protocol for the measurement of eye dominance in young children.
11. Graham Erickson. Sports Vision: Vision Care for the Enhancement of Sports Performance.
12. Ajay Kr Bhootra and Dr Sumitra. Elite Sports and Vision.
13. Lauren Taylor. Anticipation Skill in Sport.
14. Mitchell Scheiman and Bruce Wick. Clinical Management of Binocular Vision.
15. John R Griffin and J David Grisham. Binocular Anomalies: Diagnosis and Vision Therapy.
16. Geraint Griffiths. A Strategy for Sports Vision Assessment.
17. DFC Loran and CJ MacEwen. Sports Vision.
18. Emma Hilton. Exercise-eyes: Effects of exercise on ocular health.
19. Geraint Griffiths. The Incidence of Ametropia in Elite Sport.
20. Geraint Griffiths. Colour Preference – Comparative Study.
21. Donald FC Loran. Sports Eye Wear and Eye Care – A Survey of UK and US Practitioners.
22. Donald Loran and Geraint Griffiths. Visual Performance and Soccer Skills in Young Players.
23. Brian Ariel. Ocular and Systemic Health –The Role of Exercise and Nutrition.
24. Ajay Kumar Bhootra. Clinical Refraction Guide.
25. Ajay Kumar Bhootra. Basics of Computer Vision Syndrome.
26. Brendan Scott. How does altitude affect the body and why does it affect people differently? https://medicalxpress.com/news/2018-06-altitude-affect-body-people-differently.html

Index

Page numbers followed by *f* refer to figure and *t* refer to table.

C

W

Y

Z